STRENGTH TRAINING
for BEGINNERS

Previously published as STRENGTH TRAINING FOR STRONG BONES

JOAN BASSEY, PH.D., and SUSIE DINAN

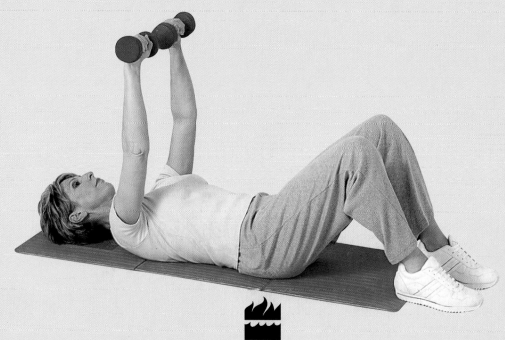

HarperResource

An imprint of HarperCollins*Publishers*

Created and produced by
Carroll & Brown Publishers
20 Lonsdale Road
Queen's Park
London NW6 6RD

Originally published in the USA by HarperCollins in 2001
as *Strength Training for Strong Bones*

Managing Editor Becky Alexander
Art Director Tracy Timson

Editorial Assistant Charlotte Beech
Designer Roland Codd

Photography Jules Selmes

Picture Credits
5 (right) Prof. P. Motta/Dept of Anatomy/University. 'La Sapienza', Rome/SPL,
54 Getty Images Stone, 60 Getty Images Stone, 62 Thomas Hart Shelby/Retna,
83 Telegraph Colour Library, 87 Getty Images Stone

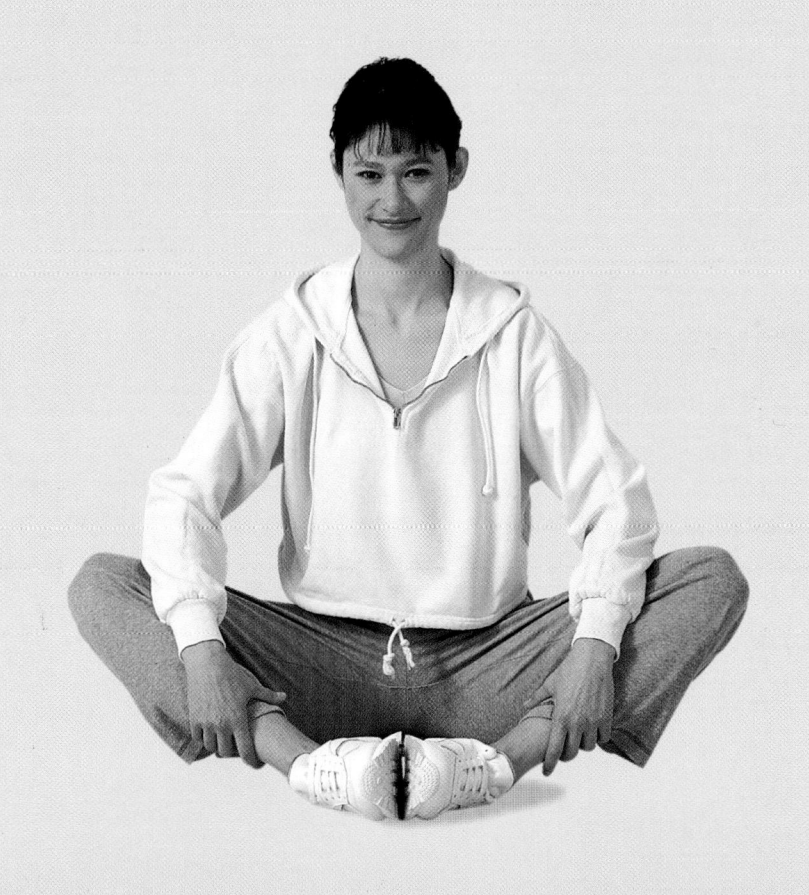

Contents

Introduction

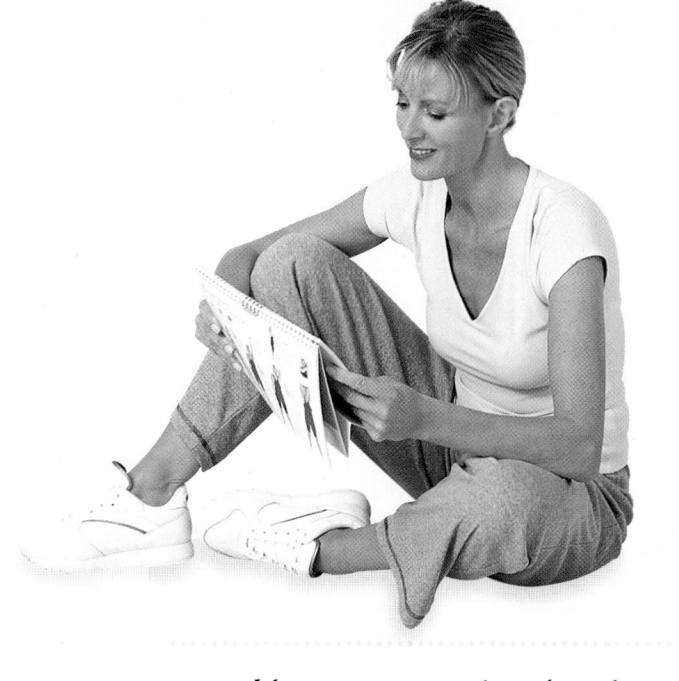

This book is designed to help healthy women adopt a lifestyle that will optimize bone strength and so reduce their risk of developing osteoporosis, or "brittle bones." Its emphasis is specifically on activities that promote bone strength and reduce the risk of fracture.

These exercises are not intended to help you lose weight (that might not be a good idea for your bones anyway) but they will improve your muscle strength and give you a more streamlined, youthful look. They should make you feel younger and more confident because your increased strength will make many physical demands and activities easier.

Research has now shown that women can take steps to prevent or manage osteoporosis, and that exercise is beneficial. The skeleton responds well to brief bouts of varied activity, which are easier to fit into a busy schedule than such exercise regimes as those aimed at reducing the risk of cardiovascular disease. The exercises within this book are easy to master and most of them can be performed at home.

How to use this book

Once you have read the introduction and discovered the importance of exercise for bone strength, turn to the section on Getting Started (page 18) and complete the questionnaires at the back of the book, which will help you to find which exercises are right for you.

Then, it's straight into the step-by-step program of exercises to do at home. This book's unique format allows you to stand it up nearby for easy reference during your exercise session. The last section "Activities for Life" explores other types of exercises and activities that you can safely incorporate into your lifestyle to complement your strong bones workout.

What is osteoporosis?

Osteoporosis has been recognized as a problem, deserving of research attention and medical treatment, since about 1980. One in three women develop osteoporosis or "brittle bone" disease. This means that bones break easily because the skeleton has become fragile.

Age-related osteoporosis is caused by gradual loss of bone mineral; this is a normal process, and is not a disease caused by infection. As bone mineral is lost, the bones do not shrink in size but become fragile and porous—"osteoporosis" means porous bone.

From mid-life onward, the skeleton slowly loses bone mineral. If this bone loss is combined with less than average bone mineral density (BMD) before the menopause, then osteoporotic fractures become increasingly likely as the years go by. However, you can off-set this loss with exercise that stimulates increased bone formation, to improve your BMD. It is never too late to take steps to reduce your risk of fracture, by making sure your lifestyle includes small amounts of regular bone-friendly physical activity and a bone-friendly diet.

The silent condition

Unfortunately, a fracture is often the first sign of osteoporosis. Osteoporotic fractures can occur very easily; changing a stiff gear in the car can be enough to break a brittle bone.

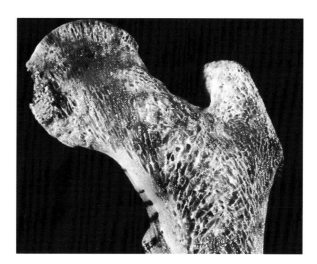

Bone structure *This is a cross-section of the top of a healthy femur showing solid outer bone and the honeycomb inside.*

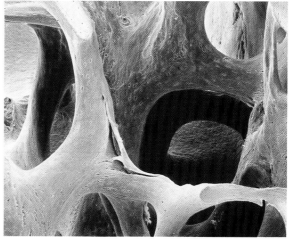

This shows the honeycomb structure magnified. If a bone becomes osteoporotic, the honeycomb walls become thinner making the bone porous and fragile.

Understanding your bones

Key facts

★ Bones should be used regularly or they will deteriorate, like muscles do if they are not used.

★ The skeleton is a support structure that is alive and responds to challenging loads.

★ The normal "loading" for the skeleton is the pull of working muscles on your bones and the force of gravity acting on your body weight. (Astronauts who live in a gravity-free environment lose bone density.)

★ Bones need a variety of brief, frequent loads every day to maintain their strength.

★ Bones need to be loaded a bit more than usual to improve their strength.

The bones that make up your skeleton are made from living tissue, which renews itself continuously throughout your life. If your skeleton is to do this effectively and remain strong, it needs regular stimulation from physical activities.

Bone is made of a calcium mineral, which gives bone its hardness and whiteness. This calcium mineral is embedded in a protein mesh of collagen, which is gristly and makes bone slightly bendy. Bone tissue is not completely solid, but has a honeycomb structure inside a thick solid outer layer. This efficient design maximizes strength, without being too heavy.

The honeycomb structure of bone provides a huge surface area which is lined with bone cells. These cells continually renew the bone substance in a systematic cycle of breakdown and re-building, called bone turnover. This process ensures that minute fractures are repaired and the bone is kept strong. This remodeling allows bone to gain strength in response to increased load, or to lose it if loads become less.

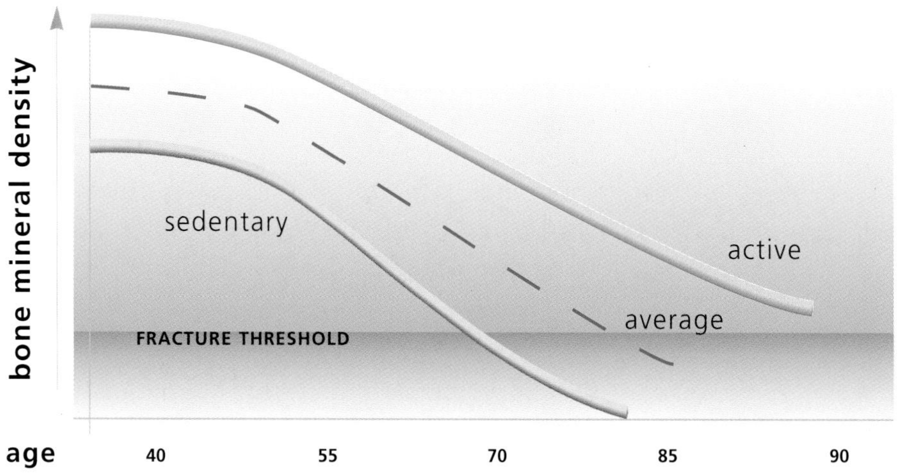

Bone changes over time This graph shows how bone mineral density (BMD) falls with age. The middle line shows the BMD of an average woman over time, and the two outer lines show the BMD of an active and sedentary woman, respectively. When BMD falls below the fracture threshold (when fracture becomes likely) a diagnosis of osteoporosis is made. The graph shows that this tends to happen at a much earlier age in sedentary women than in active women.

bone mineral density

sedentary

FRACTURE THRESHOLD

active

average

age   40   55   70   85   90

How bone changes with age

During your early years, your body accumulates bone. Up to and during adolescence, bones grow rapidly. Most of your skeleton is in place by the end of your teenage years and the consolidation of the skeleton is complete by the time you are 30 years old. It is still possible, however, to achieve improvements in BMD after this age if you change from a sedentary lifestyle to a more active one.

Some women lose very little bone as they grow older, but others can lose a lot, particularly in the first few years after the menopause because of the fall in estrogen levels that occurs when menstruation ceases. The result is a loss of bone mineral over the next few years of up to five percent each year. Fortunately, this loss later slows down to a rate of about one percent a year. Even so, the bone can eventually become so porous that fractures happen very easily. During the postmenopausal years, estrogen levels are low, and vary from one woman to another. This variation in estrogen levels may go some way toward explaining why some women are more vulnerable to osteoporosis than others.

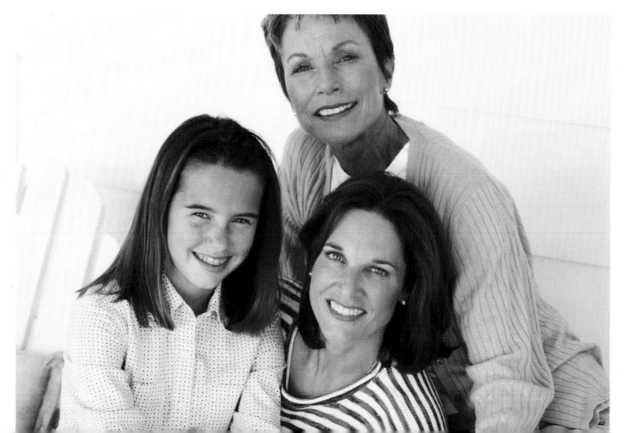

Exercise for everyone *It is never too late or too early to take care of your bones; from the age of six to sixty, physical activity will benefit your skeleton.*

Are you at risk?

There are a number of factors that increase your risk of developing osteoporosis. Many of them are genetically programmed so you cannot do anything about them, but it does help to be forewarned. There are other factors you can do something about (see pages 12–13). Your lifestyle is very important and you may need to change only a few aspects of your life to reduce your chances of developing osteoporosis. If you think you might be at risk, see your doctor to arrange a DXA bone scan and, if necessary, seek treatment to prevent fractures occurring later. The main risk factors which you cannot change are:

Gender

Women are at greater risk than men because they have smaller bones which contain less mineral. Estrogen is important for bone health in women, and estrogen levels fall at the menopause.

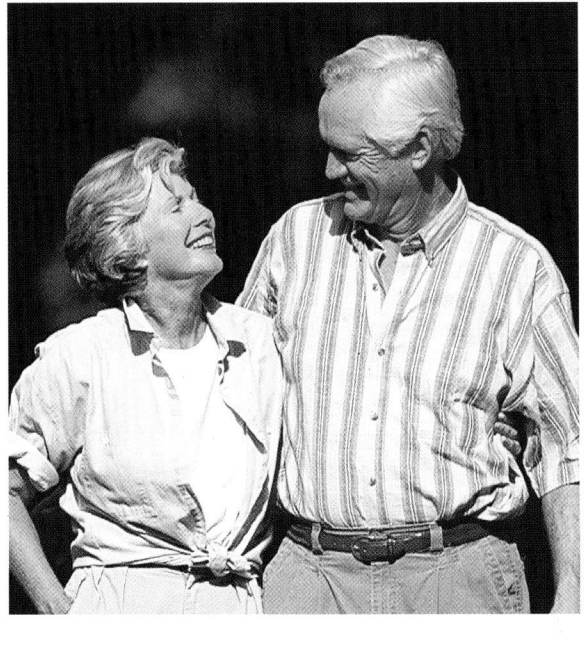

The gender divide *Women are more vulnerable to osteoporosis than men because their bones are smaller and the skeleton is not protected by testosterone.*

Family history

If you have relatives, particularly your mother or a grandmother, who have suffered from osteoporosis you are more likely to do so.

Build

Small, slight women are at greater risk than large women, because they have smaller bones and lower BMD. Women of tall, thin build are also more vulnerable because of the long thin shape of the end of their hip bone. This is where almost half of all hip fractures occur.

Early menopause or hysterectomy

Women who have stopped menstruating before 45 years of age or have had a hysterectomy (removal of the womb) before this age are at greater than average risk of developing osteoporosis. This is the case even if the ovaries were not removed. If you take hormone replacement therapy (HRT) from the time of the surgery, your risk of osteoporosis is reduced because the estrogen is replaced, but you are protected only for as long as you take HRT. Other drugs which prevent bone loss are available also.

Ethnic group

For genetic reasons, black women of African descent have a ten percent lower risk of osteoporotic fracture than white women of Caucasian descent. Asian women are somewhere in between.

Thyroid problems

Occasionally the thyroid gland becomes overactive, causing hyperactivity, or underactive, causing lethargy. It is difficult to adjust treatment to get the hormone levels exactly right. Too much thyroid hormone leads to some loss of bone.

Steroid treatment

A number of diseases are treated or managed with cortico-steroids, including rheumatoid arthritis, Crohn's disease, and severe asthma. Unfortunately, a common side effect is a weakening of the skeleton.

Gut or kidney conditions

Diseases in which absorption of calcium is difficult or too much calcium is lost in the urine threaten calcium stores and lead to loss of bone.

A history of eating disorders

Failure to eat a normal, balanced diet by young women leads to bone loss which is associated with hormonal disturbances, loss of menstrual periods, and extreme

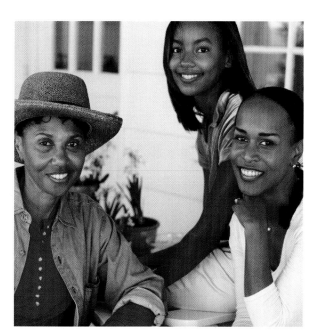

Family matters *You could be at a greater than average risk from osteoporosis if any other member of your family has a history of the condition.*

Taking the pill

Whether oral contraceptives have any effect on bones is a common concern. Contraceptive pills are a form of HRT taken to over-ride the natural pattern of hormonal release that leads to ovulation and potential pregnancy. They contain estrogen and inhibit a woman's own estrogen production. There is currently no evidence to show that taking oral contraception has long-term implications for the skeleton.

thinness. Diagnoses of osteoporosis can occur, therefore, in young women. Even after periods have resumed and body weight is back to normal, BMD may not return to previous levels. This loss of bone is likely to persist into middle age, leading to increased risk of fracture.

The weak spots

The bones that are most likely to fracture due to osteoporosis are the wrist, spine, and hip. Many of these fractures follow a fall, so maintaining good control of balance is important. You can live with fragile bones if you manage to avoid subjecting them to high impact.

Hip

Fracture of the hip is a risk for women late in life which can cause a great deal of misery. Admission to hospital and major surgery to pin the broken ends of the bone together is often needed, and although this is usually a successful operation. Many older victims never fully recover their mobility and independence.

Spine

Trying to open a stuck window or turning a key in a stiff lock can be enough to cause a vertebral fracture if your spine is osteoporotic. Signs that you might already

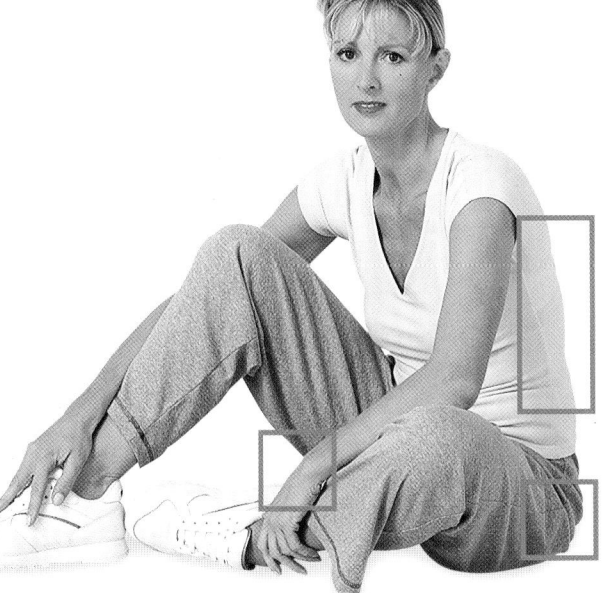

Understanding your skeleton *Certain areas of the skeleton are more at risk from fracture due to osteoporosis, namely, the hip, spine, and wrist.*

have spinal osteoporosis are height loss and curvature of the spine (also known as "Dowager's hump"). Once a vertebra has collapsed, there is, at present, no way of rebuilding it. If several vertebrae collapse, the curvature of the spine can lead to health problems. For example, respiratory diseases can develop because there is not enough room in the chest for the lungs.

Wrist

The most common cause of a fractured wrist is when you reach out and use your hand to take the impact of a fall. A broken wrist is not a disaster, but it can be very painful; it may not heal in exactly the right position and can cause long-term discomfort. A wrist fracture is a warning that you might have osteoporosis, and that it is time to take action to prevent any more serious fractures from occuring.

Don't smoke

Smoking has been shown to increase the risk of fracture, and the more cigarettes smoked each day, the greater the risk. If you smoke, then the best thing you can do for your bones is to give it up. Your skeleton will recover to some extent, and your health will benefit in many ways. Try also to avoid passive smoking.

Prevention & treatment

If you have been diagnosed with osteoporosis or think you may be at high risk, then there are a number of drugs that your doctor can prescribe. The most widely used are various forms of HRT, but other drugs have also been developed that produce similar benefits for the skeleton. You will need to discuss the options with your doctor to determine which is right for you. Since one of the major reasons for bone loss is the fall in estrogen levels after the menopause, restoring these levels with HRT prevents further loss. HRT can also increase BMD over a period of years, especially in the spine. Although HRT and other drug treatments are useful to postmenopausal women, they do not suit everyone, and there can be side effects.

The importance of exercise

Whether you choose to take a drug treatment or not, you can further improve your BMD and reduce your fracture risk by making adjustments to your lifestyle. Research has shown that women who took part in regular exercise as well as starting HRT improved their BMD more than women who either exercised only or took HRT only.

Improving bone strength The exercises contained in this book have been shown to improve BMD if practiced regularly. This exercise targets the hip (see page 50).

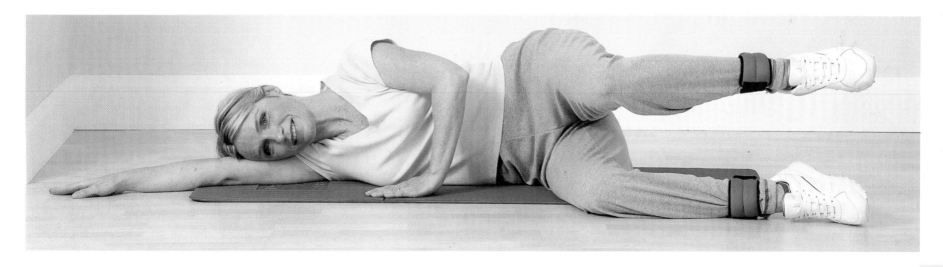

Reducing your risk

There are several steps you can take to look after your bones and to ensure that you go into the menopause in the best possible health. These steps will also help to maintain your BMD after the menopause.

Feed your bones

Because the skeleton is largely made up of calcium salts, and as it acts as a reserve for calcium (which is also vital for nerve and muscle function), it is important that your daily intake of calcium is sufficient. The recommended adequate intake (AI) is 1000 mg for women aged 31–50 and 1200 mg for those aged 51–70.

If you eat a balanced diet, you shouldn't need to take calcium supplements. But if you can't eat dairy products, or need to take a supplement for other reasons, choose one carefully: some contain more calcium than others, so compare the labels on different brands before you buy.

Vitamin D is essential for helping you to absorb calcium from your food. There are two sources of vitamin D: your diet (see right) and exposure to the sun.

Your skin can make vitamin D provided it is exposed to ultraviolet light from the sun. Half an hour three times a week of summer sun on your face and hands is recommended—this is below the amount likely to cause sunburn or skin cancer.

The amounts of vitamin D needed are small, the AI is 200 international units (IU) for women aged 19–50, and 400 IU for those over 50, and the body can build up stores which last for a few weeks. But in northern winters, the sun is too weak to be effective so it is vital to get enough in your diet. If you do not like fatty fish, then choose a supplement, but do not overdose yourself: too much is toxic.

You also need plenty of fresh fruit and vegetables which contain other vitamins and minerals essential for bone health.

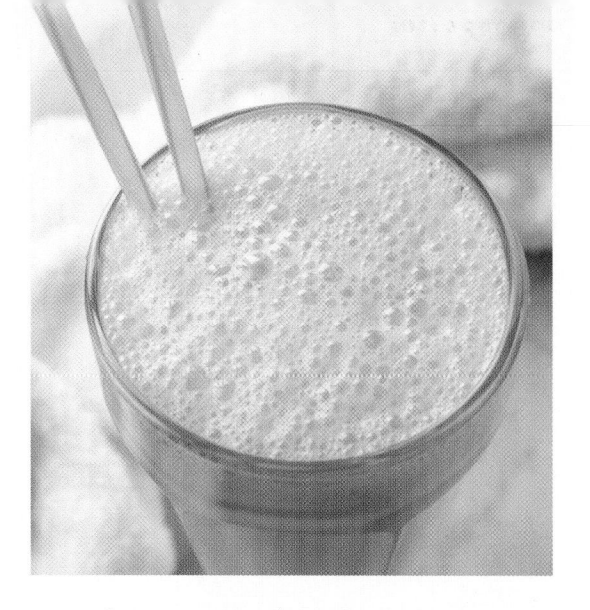

Sources of calcium and vitamin D

Calcium　The richest sources of calcium are milk, cheese, and yogurt. A quart of milk contains about 1000 mg. Dark green vegetables, almonds, and tinned sardines (if you eat the bones) also contain calcium. White bread (not brown), some brands of orange juice, and most breakfast cereals have added calcium. Mineral water can often contain calcium—but for all foods check the list on the packaging as amounts vary.

Vitamin D　Fish and seafood (salmon, tuna, herring, shrimp) are good sources, as are fish liver oils. Milk and breakfast cereals are often fortified with vitamin D.

Maintain a healthy body weight

The bigger your bones are, the stronger they are, and the heavier you are, the denser your bones are, but this is not an excuse to eat too much! It is, however, very important to realize that dieting to lose weight is not good for your bones.

Weight loss has been associated with bone loss at all ages in adult life. Women who weigh more than 150 lbs are unlikely to have an osteoporotic fracture, but clearly if you are only 5 feet tall there are health reasons why you should not weigh this much. If you are within the healthy weight limits for your height, you shouldn't go on a weight-loss diet unless your doctor recommends it.

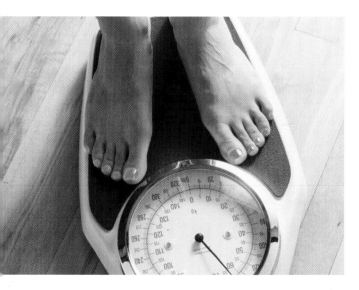

Keep an eye on the scales *The weight you carry is good for loading your bones, and any extra natural padding protects your bones from fracture if a fall occurs.*

Take some exercise

Active women have half the risk of fracture compared to those who do not take any exercise. Physical activity reduces the risk by improving both BMD and balance so that falls are less likely. Not all exercise is beneficial for your bones, however. Research has shown that the best kind of exercise for your bones is brief bouts of activity that "load" the skeleton.

Choosing the right kind of exercise

Endurance activities such as swimming or cycling are excellent forms of exercise for many reasons, but unfortunately they do not improve your bone health. Activities that provide a short sharp increase in skeletal loading are highly effective for your bones, provided they are more challenging than your normal activities (see page 94). The good news is that only a few loadings are needed to have an effect; about 50 per day. More than that does not achieve further improvement. This means that you can find time to improve your bone health without having to embark on a lengthy regimen. Regularly taking the stairs instead of the elevator might do it.

Just one minute of jumping or skipping (see pages 88–9) is useful, if it is right for you. It is important to realize, however, that these activities can prove dangerous for women with undiagnosed osteoporosis. They are therefore safe only for healthy premenopausal women.

Effective bone-loading depends on the force of gravity acting on your body, and on any weight you lift, as well as the pull of muscles on your bones as you exercise. This can be achieved in many ways and the dynamic resistance exercises in the main section of this book are safe for everyone, including older women.

Good practice

The next four pages contain advice that will help protect your spine and allow you to follow the exercises freely and safely.

The importance of posture

Everyday activities at work or at home often lead us to spend far too much time hunched over. The result is poor posture, which increases tiredness and can place a strain on the spine. Good posture is essential for the health of the skeleton and for safe and effective movement in everyday life.

Improve your posture

* ★ Lengthen your neck upward
* ★ Ease your shoulders down
* ★ Adjust your pelvic tilt
* ★ Notice you have grown taller and slimmer

Check your posture

Stand in front of a long mirror and compare yourself to the photographs (right). Ask a friend to help with this. Check often when standing or sitting, to ensure that you have not slumped down.

Bad and good posture *When you adjust your posture so that your vertebrae sit properly, you feel and look taller and slimmer. The dotted line shows how much height you gain by correcting your posture.*

Bad posture   **Good posture**

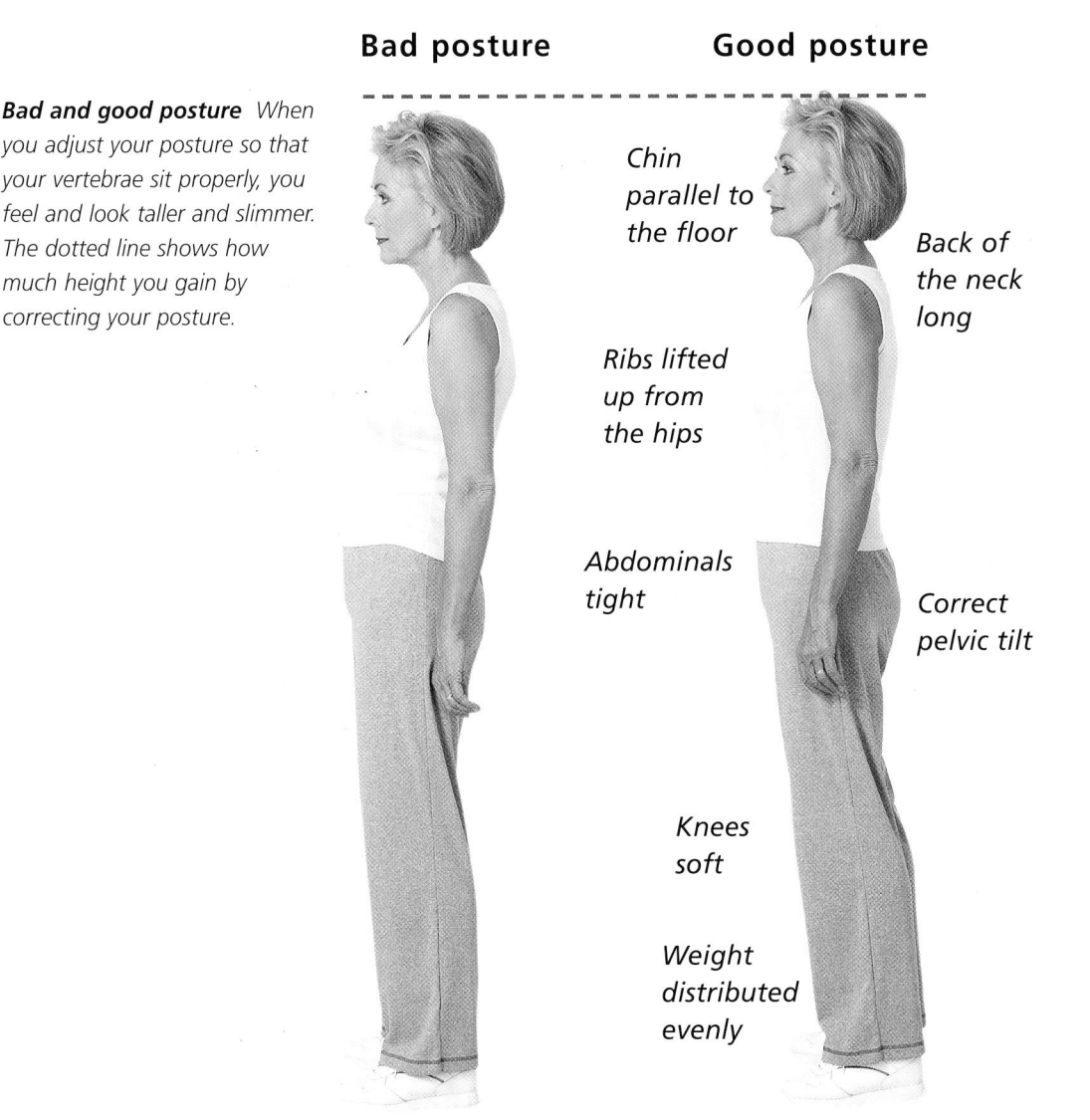

Chin parallel to the floor

Back of the neck long

Ribs lifted up from the hips

Abdominals tight

Correct pelvic tilt

Knees soft

Weight distributed evenly

The importance of pelvic tilt

A correct pelvic tilt is an essential part of good posture; the difference between the correct and incorrect position of your pelvis is a subtle one, needing only a slight tightening of some muscles such as the abdominals, and a loosening of others in your lower back. The photographs (right) show you how to achieve it.

The effect of this slight but vital adjustment is to bring your spine into alignment. Your back will still have natural curves. It should feel good but it will need practice until it becomes an automatic part of you. Do not let your abdominals tighten up so much that you cannot breathe properly.

All the exercises in the program need to be performed with a correct pelvic tilt to ensure they are done safely, accurately, and effectively.

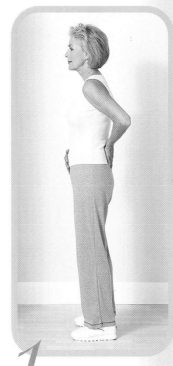

1 Stand with your feet hip-width apart and your weight distributed evenly between both feet. Relax your shoulders and place your hands as shown.

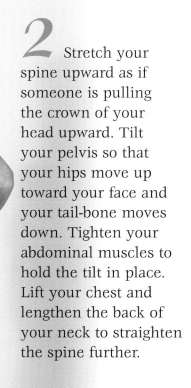

2 Stretch your spine upward as if someone is pulling the crown of your head upward. Tilt your pelvis so that your hips move up toward your face and your tail-bone moves down. Tighten your abdominal muscles to hold the tilt in place. Lift your chest and lengthen the back of your neck to straighten the spine further.

Tip

★ If you have stiff shoulders, start by shrugging your shoulders up to your ears before easing them down into position.

Look after your back

Almost everyone gets back pain at some time in their lives and it can prevent them leading an active life. One of the commonest causes of back pain is damage to the discs between the vertebrae, or a sprain of the back muscles or ligaments due to lifting something too heavy or lifting in an awkward manner.

Lifting from the floor with your arms extended and your back bent is a recipe for disaster as the leverage is poor, so the weight borne by your back is perhaps ten times the weight you are trying to lift. If the muscles are not strong enough, the ligaments take too much strain and may tear. Using the lifting technique shown here will help to protect your back; remember to use this technique for all lifting tasks.

Maintaining good posture throughout the day and using a chair that supports your lower back helps to prevent back pain. If you have a back problem or have had a hip fracture, you should avoid lifting heavy objects.

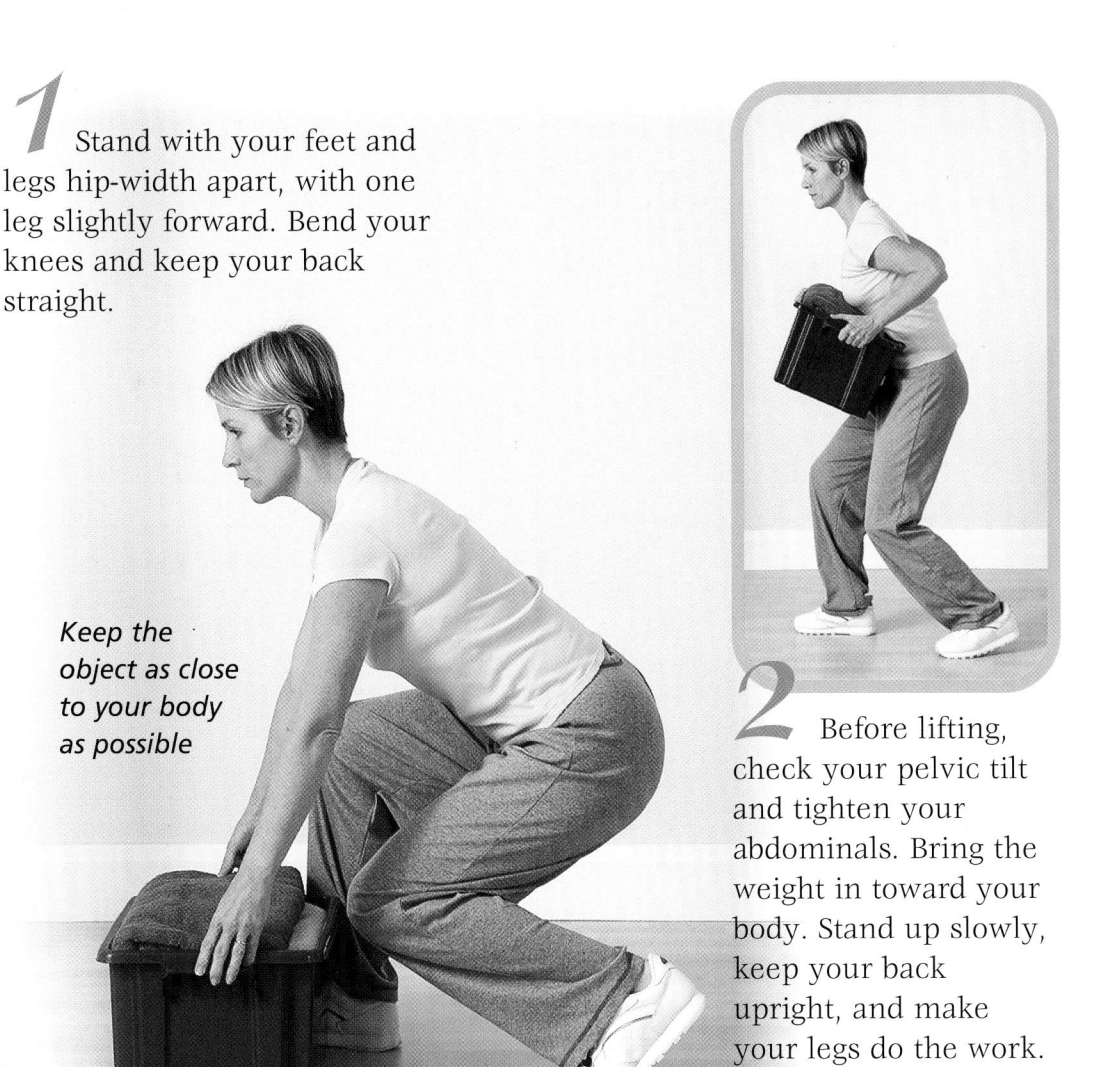

1 Stand with your feet and legs hip-width apart, with one leg slightly forward. Bend your knees and keep your back straight.

Keep the object as close to your body as possible

2 Before lifting, check your pelvic tilt and tighten your abdominals. Bring the weight in toward your body. Stand up slowly, keep your back upright, and make your legs do the work.

Strengthen your pelvic floor muscles

Many women become less active than they would like to be because they suffer from weak pelvic floor muscles. These muscles help control the bladder outlet and they are often weakened or damaged during childbirth. The embarrassing result of this is that urine leaks out easily. Like any muscles, pelvic floor muscles grow weaker with age, but they will improve in strength if exercised regularly.

Pelvic floor exercises

If you are out of practice with your pelvic floor muscles, you will need to rediscover them. Try the exercises seated to begin with. You will find the muscles easier to locate in this position and if the rest of your body is relaxed. When you have mastered the exercises you can do them any time, anywhere, because nobody but you will know what you are doing. If you have weak pelvic floor muscles, do both exercises four times a day until there is an improvement, then a minumum of once a day for maintenance.

1 Slow Close, and draw up the back, then the front passages in your pelvic floor area as slowly and as strongly as you can, as if you were trying to prevent passing wind and urine. The feeling is one of "squeeze in and lift up." Hold for a count of 6, then release slowly, and with control. Repeat 4 times.

2 Fast In one swift movement, tighten and lift both the back and front passages in the pelvic floor area. Hold for a count of one, then release slowly, and with control. Repeat 6 times.

Caution

★ Avoid tightening your abdominals or buttocks, squeezing your legs together, or holding your breath.

★ Do not practice these exercises while urinating as this may cause infection.

Getting started

This section sets out guidelines to ensure you get maximum benefit from the Home Exercises (see page 36) and the recommended Activities for Life (see page 80). The guidelines are linked to two questionnaires (see pages 92–5) which you must complete. These assess your current health and level of physical activity and will enable you to tailor your own exercise prescription. Everyone is different so it is important to choose the exercises that are right for you.

Starting points

Everyone has different amounts of activity in their lives already. If you are regularly active you may need to add only one or two bone-specific exercises to your routine depending on what kind of exercise you are already doing. To get this right, find out where you are starting from with the physical activity questionnaire on page 94. If you are totally sedentary and unused to

Before you start

★ Do not exercise on a day that you feel unwell or very tired.

★ Wear appropriate footwear and comfortable clothing, ideally cotton.

★ Ensure the room is clear of obstructions, not too hot or cold, and well ventilated.

★ Make sure you will not be interrupted.

exercise, this book is for you too. The good practice section and these guidelines will enable you to tackle the Home Exercises one by one, sensibly and safely.

Health issues

Some of the exercises will be more suitable for you than others, so before you start the program, complete the health questionnaire on page 92. This will help you to select the most beneficial combination of exercises and makes it

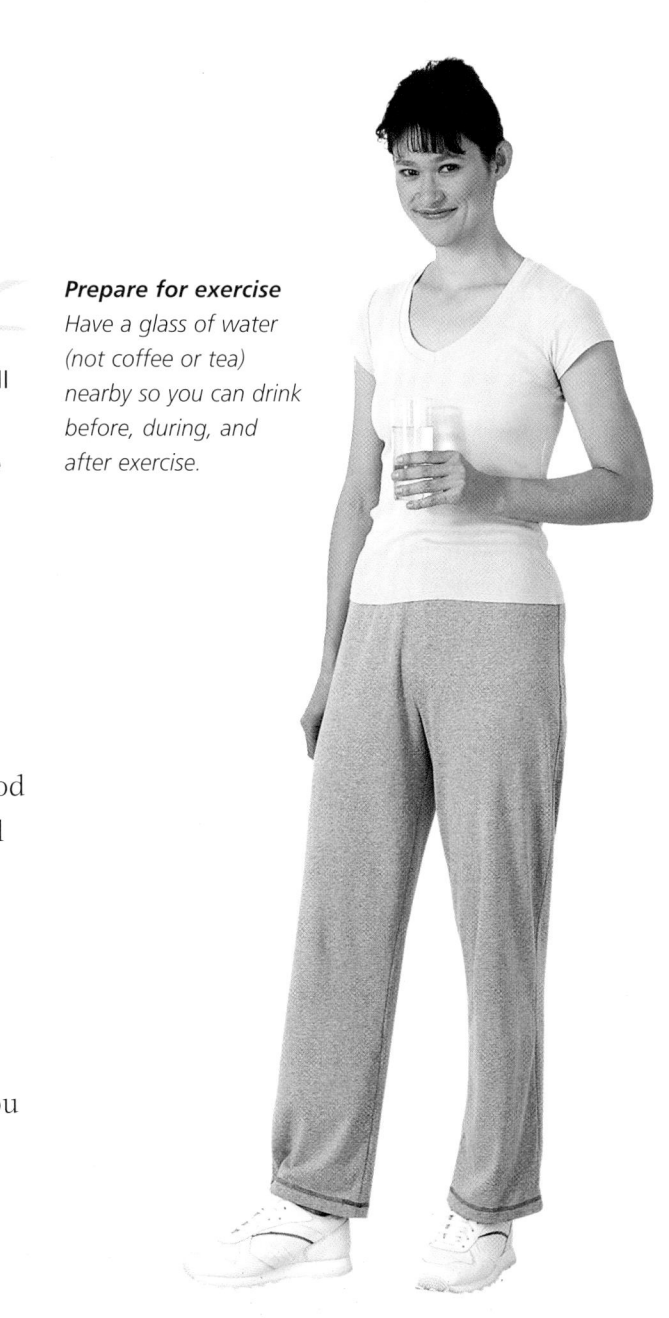

Prepare for exercise
Have a glass of water (not coffee or tea) nearby so you can drink before, during, and after exercise.

clear whether or not you should check with your doctor before getting started. This book has been written with healthy adult women aged up to 70 years in mind.

Setting goals

We all need goals to keep us going. Think about what you want to achieve, plan your program and chart your progress using the

Getting the most from exercise

★ Always warm up and cool down.

★ Take pride in using the correct technique.

★ Move with control and good posture.

★ Always work at your own level and progress cautiously.

★ Never exercise to the point of exhaustion.

★ Progress each exercise week by week to maintain the load on the skeleton and ensure you get an improvement.

★ Work through all the recommended stages of progression.

★ Avoid trying to beat the clock or another person. This program is not about winning, it is about long-term benefit.

questionnaire on page 94. Your own motivation is essential. Your bones need regular exercise for the rest of your life, not over-enthusiastic bursts of physical activity at intervals.

★ Set aside a specific time to exercise, depending on whether you are a morning or evening person, e.g. at 1.00 pm on Mondays, Wednesdays, and Saturdays.

★ Make sure your program will fit in with your daily life.

★ If you have not exercised for a long time, set yourself realistic goals and start at a leisurely pace.

★ Build up your program over time, perhaps adding a new exercise once a month.

★ If you are very short of time, do some of the exercises once a week for maintenance; this is better than doing none at all.

Listen to your body

It is important to appreciate the difference between working hard and over-working. If you are working effectively, you should

Warning signs

★ Stop exercising and seek medical advice if you experience:
  Pain or discomfort
  Dizziness, faintness, or nausea
  Shortness of breath
  Rapid heart rate
  Excessive sweating
  Sudden feeling of exhaustion or weakness

★ Slow down if you are:
  Feeling heavy limbed or shaky
  Breathing heavily
  Feeling overheated
  Losing concentration

be breathing a little more heavily than usual, feeling warm, perhaps sweating lightly, and you should have a sensation of effort in your muscles.

Pain of any kind is a warning sign so never ignore or work through it. If any pain persists when you stop exercising, seek medical advice.

Getting the load up

Most of the exercises depend on the resistance caused by the pull of gravity on your body mass. Some need the addition of weights or other simple equipment to increase the resistance. This is why we refer to "weight-training." Weights have advantages for bone-loading because of the stabilizing muscle activity needed around the spine and hip and the variety of loading. However, they are potentially dangerous if dropped or if your lift gets out of control, so set an upper limit of 15 lbs for arm lifts and 25 lbs for leg lifts. Some exercises carry lower limits for safety; look for them under "progression." Take care when moving weights around. A few exercises require a partner; if you arrange to do them with a friend it will help you to stick to your routine.

Daily half dozen

★ Practice good posture and pelvic tilt throughout the day (see pages 14–15).

★ Do lots of pelvic floor exercises (see page 17).

★ Do one balance exercise. Vary them from day to day (see pages 38–43).

★ Go for a brisk five minute walk.

★ Climb a few flights of stairs.

★ Do some stretches (see pages 78–9).

Weekly program

★ Aim for three 40 minute sessions a week. Choose exercises that address your current needs from among the Home Exercises (see page 36) or the Activities for Life (see page 80). There are suggestions on page 95.

★ You may wish to target your hip or wrist if you have below normal BMD at that site, so we have identified the specific benefits of each exercise in the Purpose boxes on each page.

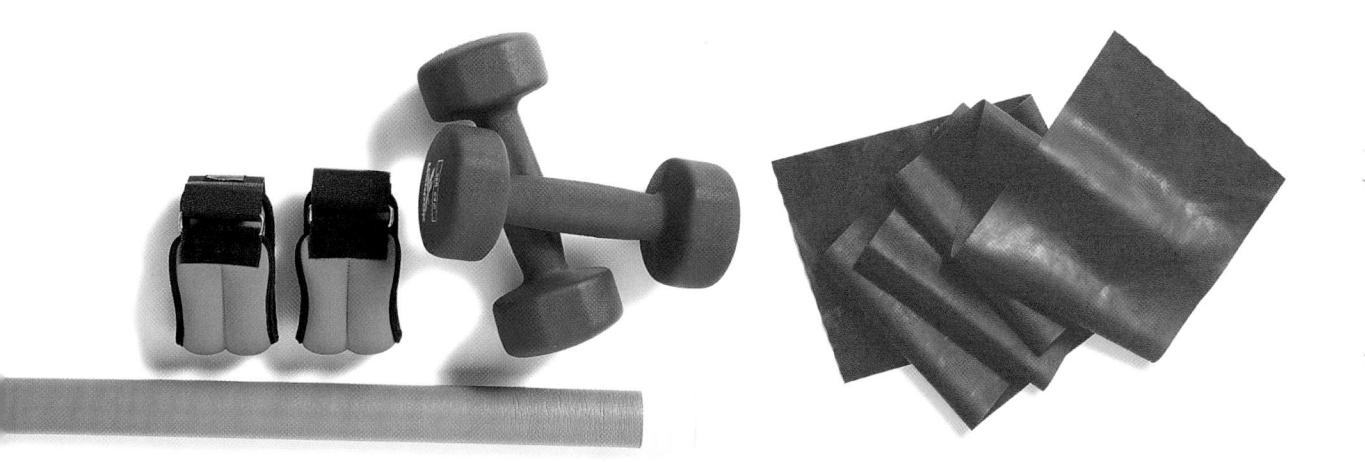

Equipment to increase the resistance *Comfortable, covered strap-on weights, dumbbells, and body bars are available from all leading suppliers of exercise equipment. They come in graded sets from 1lb upward.*

Wide strips of strong rubber material, known as resistance bands, are also available in various color-coded thicknesses. They give you a graded resistance to work against as you try to stretch them out.

Balance as well as bone-loading

Postural stability can be improved with practice. This will help to protect you from falls which is especially important if you already have fragile bones.

The benefits for bone

The exercises are effective for increasing BMD because they cause your muscles to generate large forces in the tendons which attach them to bone. The exercises have been chosen because they were found in research studies to benefit bone at the sites which are most liable to fracture. If you do these exercises in the way they are prescribed, three times a week, they will probably increase your BMD by three or four percent over a year, and if you are post-menopausal, they will at least prevent further bone loss. Some women have shown increases of up to ten percent and those with the lowest BMD are the most likely to benefit.

Commitment

Bone changes slowly, so a long-term commitment is needed. Do a little exercise regularly and choose activities that you enjoy so that you will want to continue. Variety is good for your bones and helps to prevent boredom. Do not despair if the exercises take ages to do at first; you will get quicker with practice. Just like muscle, bone will deteriorate again if you stop exercising and your gains will slowly be lost.

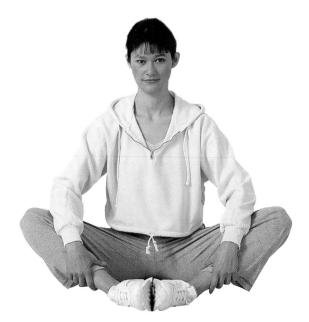

Stretch and relaxation

Always rest in between bouts of exercise; there is no need to get out of breath or tired. Stretching after you have exercised is effective for keeping you supple.

Warming up

The circulation, mobility, and stretching exercises on the next few pages are essential preparation for the main program. These gentle, rhythmic movements, mobilizers, and held stretches get your muscles, joints, and reflexes awake, loosened up, warm, and ready for action. Stretching is especially important if you have been sitting for a while as your muscles may have become slightly stiff. Working through the warming up section will help to ensure that you do not injure yourself, and you will find the main program more comfortable to perform.

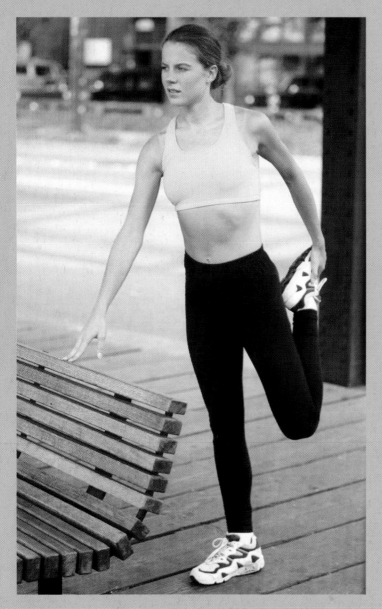

THE BENEFITS OF WARM-UP

Muscles work most effectively when they are warm. They can generate more power and are stronger than when they are cold. Although you may be indoors and do not actually feel cold, your leg and arm muscles are likely to be at a lower temperature than your trunk. For example, if you feel your calf muscle, you may find that the skin feels cooler than the skin on your neck. If you sit outdoors in cold weather, you may find that it is more difficult to walk when you stand up; this is because your leg muscles have been allowed to cool down in order to conserve heat and energy for the rest of the body.

When you begin to exercise, it takes a few minutes before your blood flow increases and enough heat is generated to adjust your muscle temperature. You get hot when you exercise, but only after you have been exercising for a while. The warm-up exercises are designed to get your body ready before you start the main program.

Walk, side-step, & march

Purpose

Circulation exercises, sometimes referred to as pulse-raisers, are low-intensity, rhythmical activities that get the large muscle groups of your arms and legs moving to boost their supply of oxygen-rich blood and warm them up.

This is the start of your program, so make it fun. Put on some lively music, and enjoy the exercises. Starting your workout in this way can release tension, improve your focus, and motivate you for the exercises to come.

Your movements should be gentle, and your breathing should be steady. Build up the size and pace of your moves gradually; this allows the heart rate to increase steadily, making for safer, and more effective exercise.

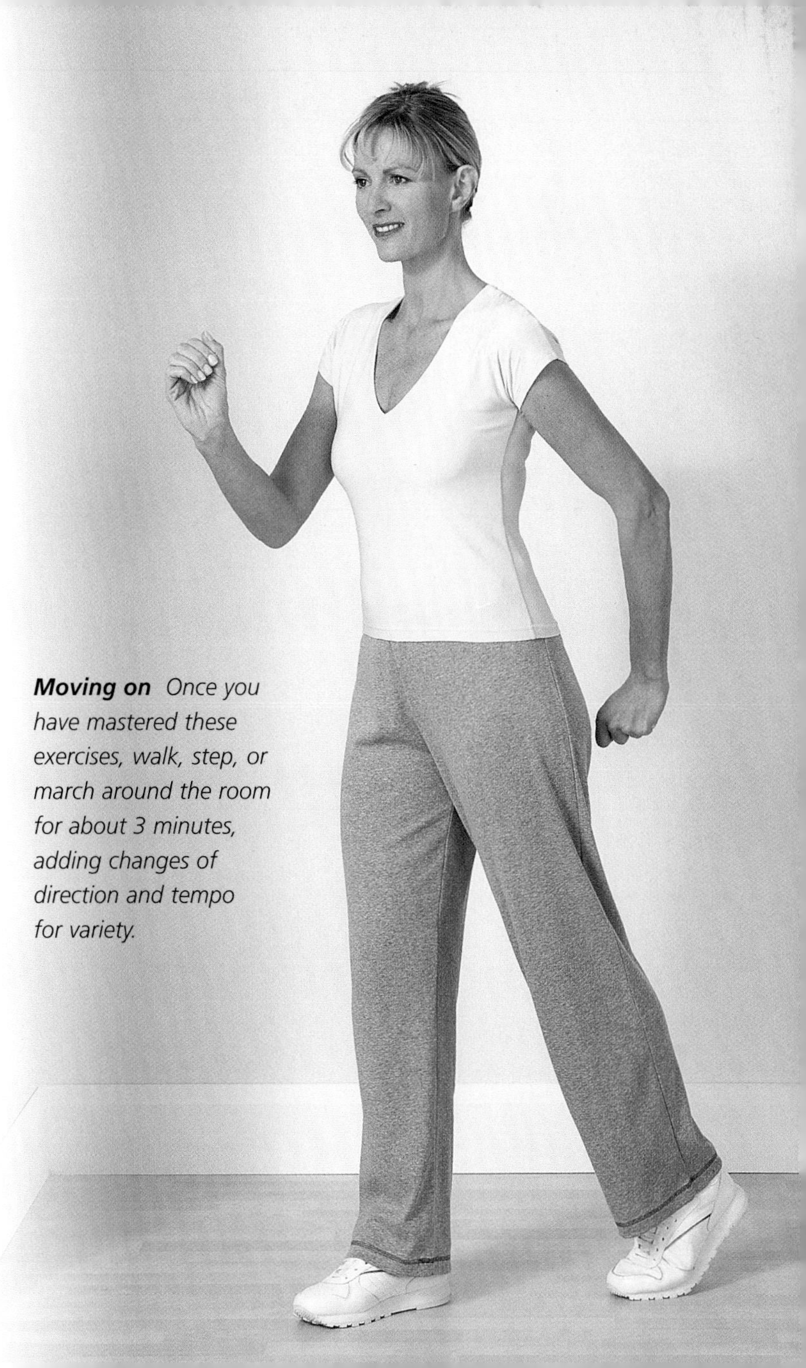

Moving on *Once you have mastered these exercises, walk, step, or march around the room for about 3 minutes, adding changes of direction and tempo for variety.*

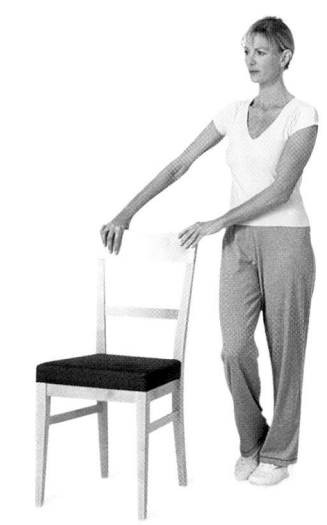

Adaptation

To help you balance, you can perform the side-step exercise holding onto a chair.

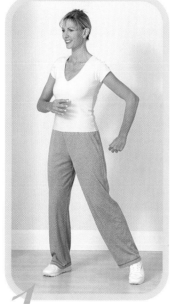

1 Walk Check your pelvic tilt, and tighten your abdominals. Walk on the spot, keeping your toes on the floor. Lift your arms with each step. Continue for 2 minutes.

1 March March gently on the spot, lifting the opposite arm to the lifted knee. Continue for 2 minutes.

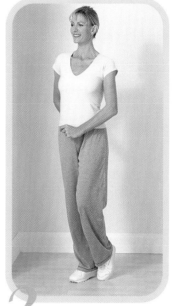

1 Side-step Step to the side, transferring your weight from the ball to the heel of your foot.

2 Bring your other foot in to touch the floor. Repeat to the other side. Swing your arms in the direction of the step. Continue for 2 minutes.

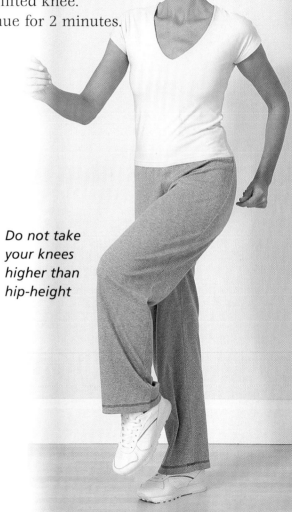

Do not take your knees higher than hip-height

Shoulder & ankle mobilizers

To perform everyday actions with ease and comfort, freely moving shoulder joints are essential. Tasks such as reaching a high shelf or serving at tennis can be difficult if you have stiff shoulder joints.

Take time and care to explore your full range of movement in each direction. Move your shoulders forward, up, back, and down. Stop immediately if you feel any discomfort. Careful control and concentration on the quality of movement will improve your technique, and increase your enjoyment and body-awareness.

When combined with good posture, this exercise can give your shoulder line and upper body a great shape. Slow shoulder circles are also a great way to release tension in the shoulder muscles; this is an area where many people carry tension.

Mobile ankles ensure good balance, as the joints can respond better to uneven surfaces.

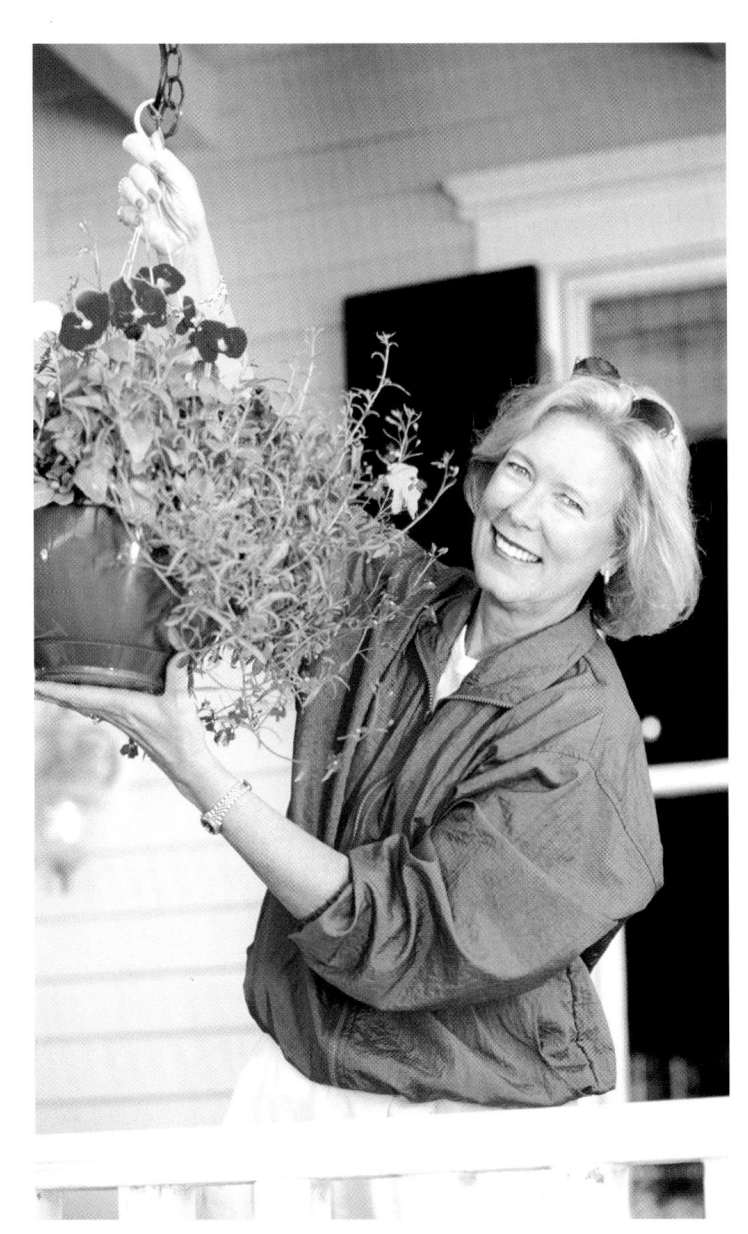

Stay strong and active *Supple shoulder joints and strong shoulder muscles are vital for maintaining your reach, and allowing you to lift heavy items like this hanging basket from shoulder height.*

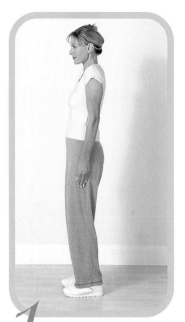

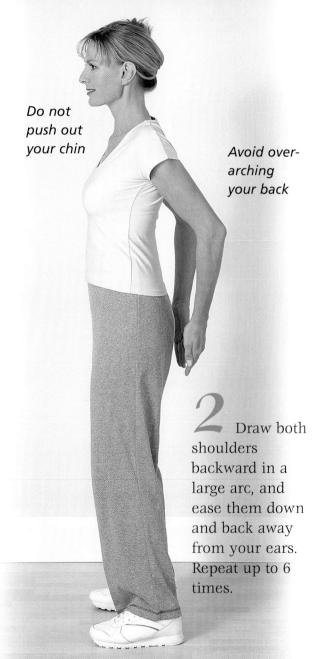

Do not push out your chin

Avoid over-arching your back

1 Shoulder Stand tall with your feet and legs a little wider than hip-width apart. Relax your shoulders and allow your arms to rest by your sides. Check your pelvic tilt and tighten your abdominals. Take both shoulders forward, then lift them up to your ears.

2 Draw both shoulders backward in a large arc, and ease them down and back away from your ears. Repeat up to 6 times.

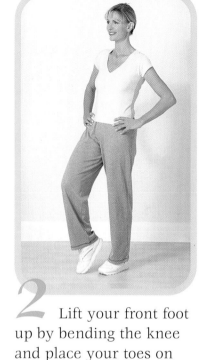

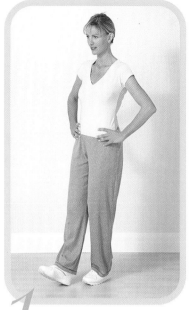

1 Ankle Stand tall, check your pelvic tilt, and tighten your abdominals. Transfer your weight to one leg, and place your other heel forward.

2 Lift your front foot up by bending the knee and place your toes on the floor. Repeat this action 6 times. Repeat with the other foot.

Common mistake

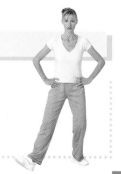

★ Avoid taking your feet too far apart as this reduces your range of movement in the ankle, and puts unnecessary strain on the supporting leg.

Side & twist: spine mobilizers

Purpose

These exercises help to mobilize the spine, maintain its range of movement, and reduce the risk of back injury when you exercise.

M obility exercises stimulate the release of synovial fluid, the joints' natural "oil"; this fluid nourishes, lubricates, and protects your joint structures. They also help to keep the vulnerable intervertebral discs protected.

A supple spine absorbs impact more efficiently than a stiff spine. These exercises take the spine joint through their full range of movement in two directions, which are often neglected.

It is very important that you maintain a correct pelvic tilt for spine exercises. Move slowly, fluently, and with control. Extend the spine to its full natural range, but never to the point of discomfort. Take a moment as you come back to center each time to lengthen the spine and check your posture.

Caution

★ Bear in mind that each individual's range of movement is different, so although you need to get your position as close to the pictures as possible, it is important also that you find the movement comfortable.

Adaptation

If you experience any pain in your lower back, or if you find it difficult to rotate without moving your hips, do the Twist exercise seated. Remember to do a pelvic tilt before you start.

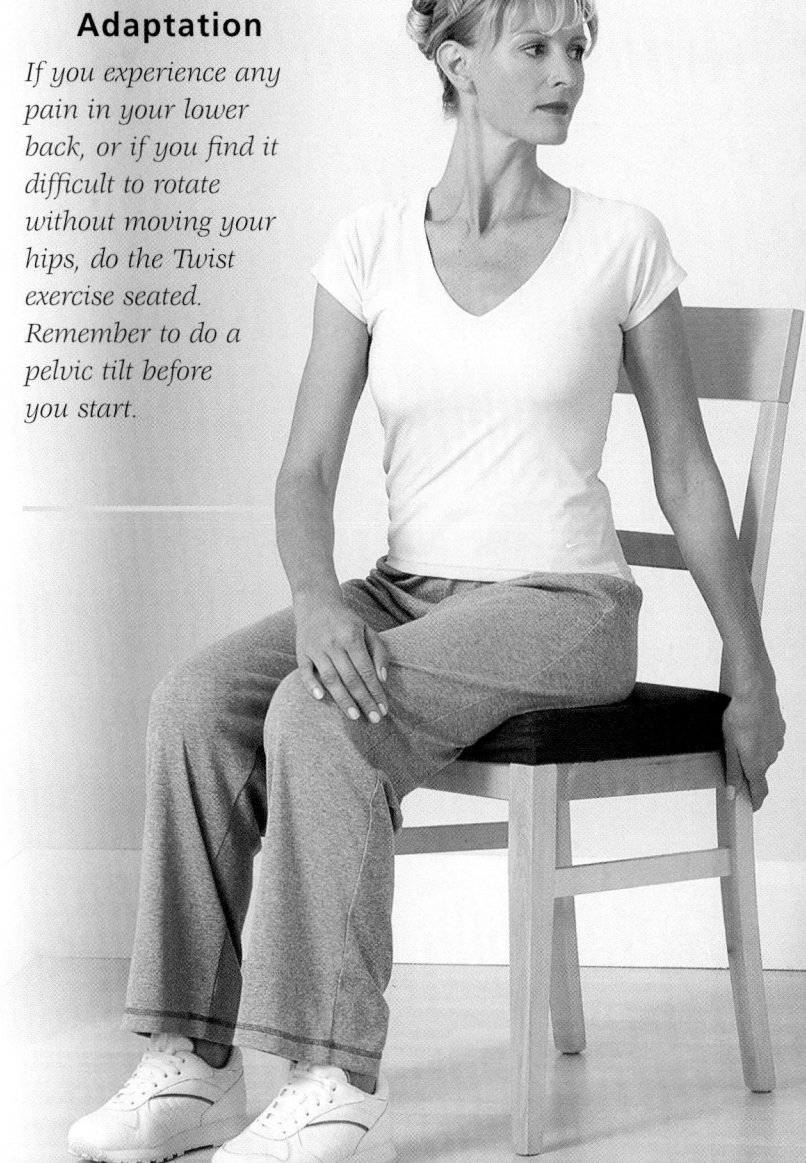

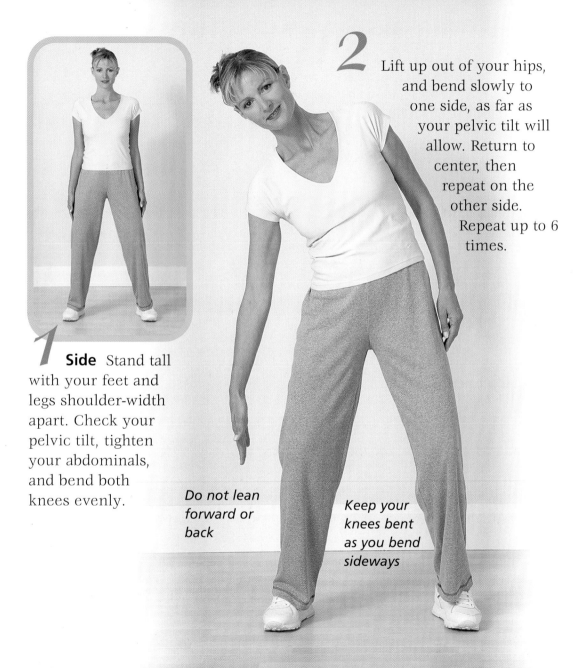

2 Lift up out of your hips, and bend slowly to one side, as far as your pelvic tilt will allow. Return to center, then repeat on the other side. Repeat up to 6 times.

Do not lean forward or back

Keep your knees bent as you bend sideways

1 Side Stand tall with your feet and legs shoulder-width apart. Check your pelvic tilt, tighten your abdominals, and bend both knees evenly.

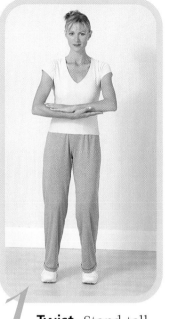

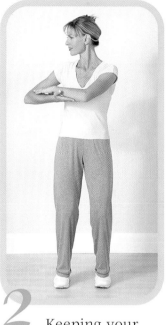

1 Twist Stand tall with your feet and legs hip-width apart. Check your pelvic tilt, tighten your abdominals, and bend both knees evenly. Hold your arms at chest height, resting one on top of the other.

2 Keeping your hips, knees, and feet facing forward, lengthen your spine, and slowly turn your upper body and head to one side, as far as you can. Return to center, then repeat on the other side. Repeat up to 6 times.

Calf & thigh stretches

Purpose

These stretches prepare muscles for the exercises to follow, and help to maintain the range of movement in the ankle and hip joints.

Muscles are adaptable and make themselves shorter over time if they are continually in a shortened position. This frequently happens to the calf muscle in women who do not wear flat shoes or walk barefoot. Such shortened calf muscles restrict ankle movements, but regular stretching reduces the stiffness and improves mobility.

Similarly, lengthening the quadriceps (the four muscles at the front of the thigh) through stretching improves the range of movement at the hip, transforms posture, and so can help to prevent or alleviate back problems. Even if you have good posture, use a wall to support yourself, so you can focus fully on the quality of your stretch.

Stretching the quadriceps is one of the most important ways of counteracting the effects of prolonged sitting. Given today's sedentary lifestyles, both at work and home, this is a must for us all if we are to avoid becoming chair-shaped!

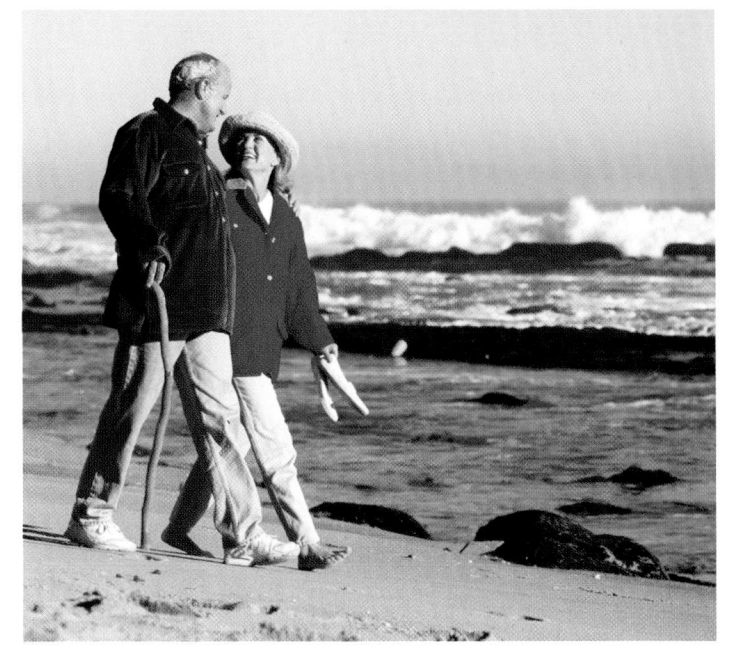

Walking barefoot *This is beneficial for the calf muscles and ankle mobility, and helps to improve your balance, so take off your shoes whenever you can.*

Adaptation

If you find balance difficult, use a chair to do the calf stretch. Keep your back straight, your chest lifted, and pull your toe up toward your knee.

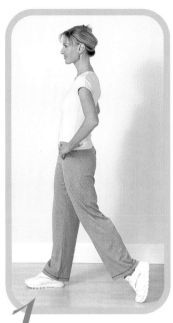

2 Bend your front knee so that it is directly above your ankle. Press your back heel onto the floor and straighten this leg until you can feel a stretch in your calf. Hold for a count of 8. Repeat with the other leg.

Lean slightly forward and upward to maintain a good body position

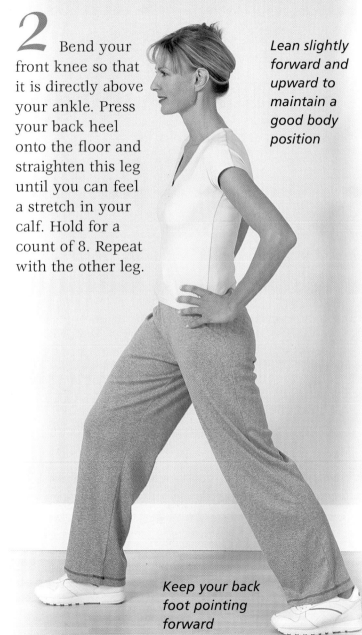

1 **Calf** Stand tall with your feet and legs hip-width apart and place your hands on your hips. Check your pelvic tilt and tighten your abdominals. Keeping your toes facing forward, take a stride backward with one foot, and place it on the floor.

Keep your back foot pointing forward

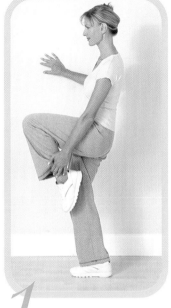

1 **Thigh** Stand tall with a hand on a wall. Check your pelvic tilt, and lift your outer knee. Take hold of your ankle.

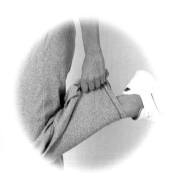

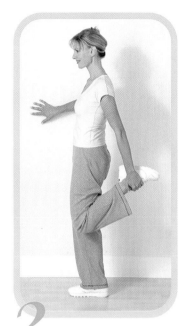

2 Take your leg backward until your knee is just behind your hip. Straighten the supporting leg then increase your pelvic tilt, and tighten your abdominals. Hold for a count of 8. Repeat with the other leg.

If you have difficulty reaching your ankle, hold your sock or pant leg.

Side & chest stretches

Purpose

To stretch the muscles in the side of your torso and across the front of your chest. Both help to maintain good posture.

Common mistake

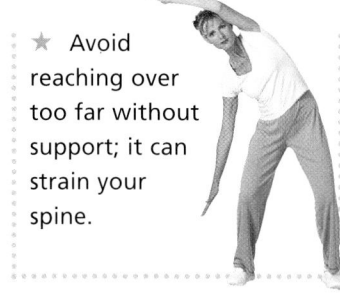

★ Avoid reaching over too far without support; it can strain your spine.

Stretching the muscles at the side of your trunk helps to maintain spinal mobility and improve your posture. It is also good for releasing tension, and this exercise will help maintain the range of movement in your shoulders. Always alternate sides when performing exercises that focus on the spine, as this gives a feeling of harmony, and keeps the spine aligned and the body symmetrical.

Stretching the pectoral muscles across the front of the chest is an uplifting activity in every way. Most of us experience some rounding of the shoulders when sitting at a desk or because of poor posture, and with this comes a sagging of the chest and restricted breathing. Pectoral stretches transform your posture as they lift the shoulders up and back, and in so doing, strengthen your upper back. This opens out your chest, and allows for deeper breathing.

The positioning of your arms needs particular care when doing the side stretch.

Adaptation

If balance is a problem, do the Side Stretch seated. Remember to check your pelvic tilt before you start.

1 Side Stand tall with your feet shoulder-width apart. Check your pelvic tilt and tighten your abdominals. Place one hand on your hip, and lift the other upward.

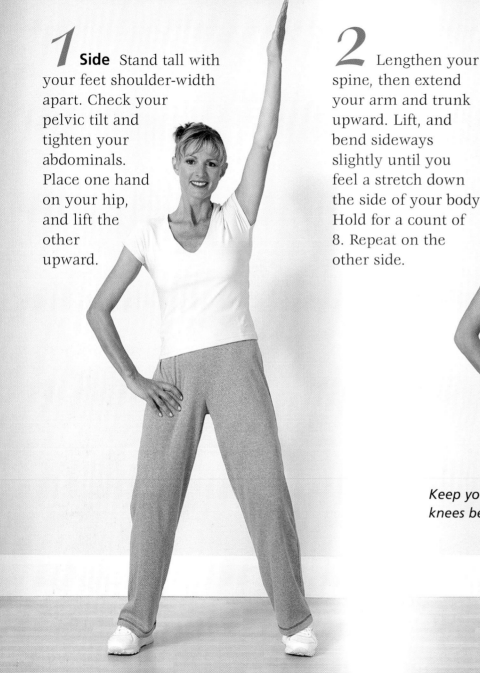

2 Lengthen your spine, then extend your arm and trunk upward. Lift, and bend sideways slightly until you feel a stretch down the side of your body. Hold for a count of 8. Repeat on the other side.

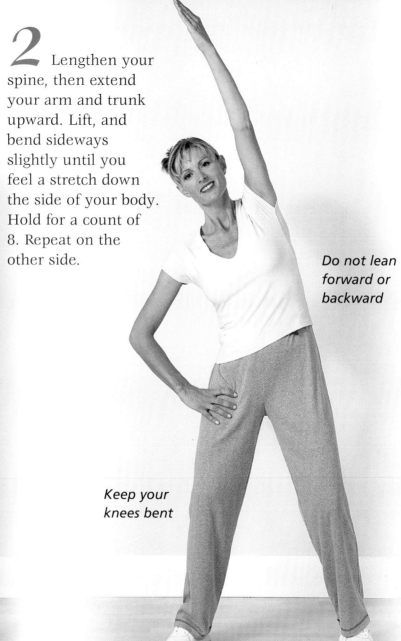

Do not lean forward or backward

Keep your knees bent

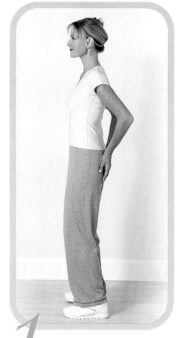

1 Chest Stand tall with your feet and legs hip-width apart. Place your hands on your bottom. Check your pelvic tilt and tighten your abdominals. Lengthen your spine, lift your chest, and take both elbows back until you feel a stretch across your chest. Hold for a count of 8.

Hamstring & **tricep** stretches

The group of muscles located along the back of your thighs (the hamstrings) are among the most neglected muscles in the body, as well as the most compromised by an inactive lifestyle. Shortened, tight hamstrings can lead to restricted movement and back problems, as well as an increased risk of injury.

The hamstrings may be notoriously tight muscles but they also respond well to attention, and progress will be felt swiftly. Stretching these muscles can give you a new lease of life as many actions become easier.

The triceps muscles are located along the back of your arm. Stretching them will ensure suppleness in the shoulder joints so that upward reaching movements can be managed with ease.

Active lifestyle *Regular stretching can improve the performance of your muscles, during both sport and everyday activities.*

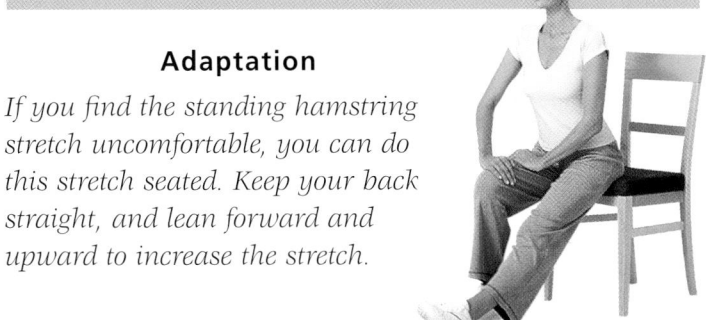

Adaptation

If you find the standing hamstring stretch uncomfortable, you can do this stretch seated. Keep your back straight, and lean forward and upward to increase the stretch.

1 Hamstring Stand tall with your feet and legs hip-width apart. Check your pelvic tilt and tighten your abdominals. Lengthen your spine and transfer your weight to one leg. Slide your other foot forward, keeping your foot on the floor.

Keep your chest lifted

Ensure your hips are level as you stretch

2 Place both hands at the top of your weighted leg. Bend this knee as you bend forward from the hips until you feel a stretch in the back of your straight leg. Hold for a count of 8. Repeat with the other leg.

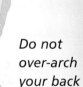

1 Tricep Stand tall as before with your knees bent slightly. Place one hand on your shoulder and take the other arm across your chest. Check your pelvic tilt and tighten your abdominals.

Keep the spine and neck long

Do not over-arch your back

2 Ease your raised arm up and back until you feel a stretch in your underarm. Aim to get the fingertips of your raised arm between your shoulder blades. Hold for a count of 8. Repeat with the other arm.

Home exercises

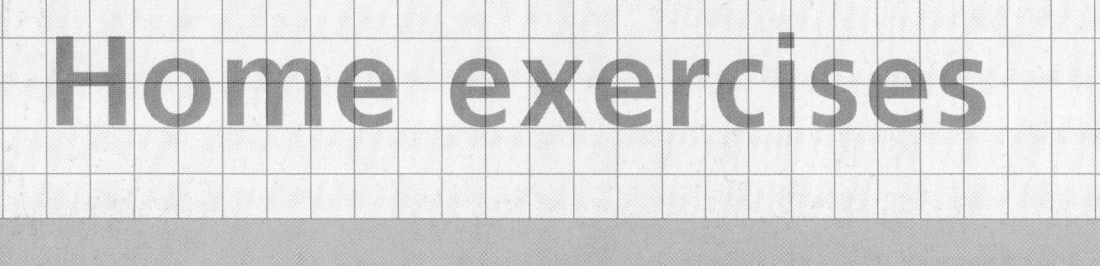

This is a series of back, leg, and arm exercises to load your skeleton in ways that should optimize your BMD. There are also balance exercises to help reduce your risk of falls. Between them these exercises will reduce your risk of fracture. The top pages include cautions for your safety and advice about how to progress. The bottom pages give detailed step-by-step instructions for each exercise. Invest time at the beginning paying careful attention to these instructions so that you master the correct technique and become competent quickly. With each new exercise, allow two sessions to learn the movement pattern, using the easiest alternative, before you begin to train in earnest.

Some of the bone loading exercises form complete packages, which have been evaluated as such in research trials; they may be effective only if practiced together. One package is the first six leg exercises (pages 48–59) and the other package is the Arm Press (page 66), All-fours (page 72), and the Wrist Press, Twist, & Pull (page 74).

A WORK-OUT FOR YOUR BONES

For improvement in BMD with weight-training, you need to lift at least 70 percent of your maximum. This level is best tested in a gym (see page 87) but you can judge it at home from the effort you apply. If the eighth lift is easy you're below 70 percent; if you can only just manage the last few lifts, you're above 80. You should train three times a week.

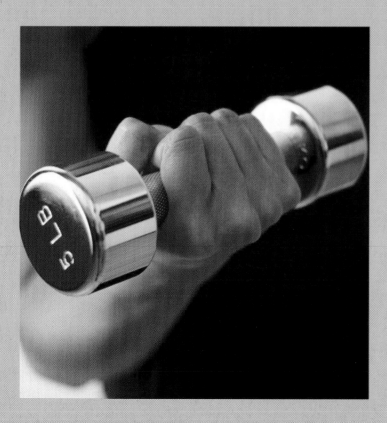

For maintenance of bone strength, continue to train once a week at the level you achieved. This should at least prevent further bone loss, which is a benefit if you are postmenopausal because these years are associated with progressive bone loss. When you are ready to use weights:

★ Follow the weight-training guidelines (right)
★ Begin with 1 lb
★ Progress in 1 lb stages
★ Use no more than 15 lbs for arm lifts
★ Use no more than 25 lbs for leg lifts.

Free weights are hard to control so the upper limits are set for safety not as a maximum for bone-loading. A larger woman will be able to lift more than a smaller one so we cannot prescribe a maximum. Few women will reach the safety limits, but if you do, then progress to a gymnasium and use the weight stacks, which allow you to use bigger weights with safety (see pages 86–7). Always move slowly, especially as you lower; you are more powerful when you move slowly and this will load the bones better.

Lift on the right and left sides in turn for all the leg exercises except the side leg lift and the leg press. If you are using weights, put one on each limb before you begin the exercise.

Weight-training

★ For each exercise aim to do 8 lifts, resting for a second between each lift.

★ Train up to 3 sets of 8 lifts (24 lifts), resting for a minute between each set.

★ Do not hold your breath; slowly count out loud to 3 as you lift (hold for a second) and to 3 as you lower.

★ When the 8th lift is no longer a challenge, it is time to progress.

★ Aim to progress every 2 weeks.

★ If you have to stop due to illness, start again with less weight.

★ Stop if you feel any pain and reduce the weight.

★ Do not over-train; up to an hour every other day is enough.

Flamingo swing

Good balance is important because if you lose your balance and fall, you might break any fragile bones. Taking steps to improve your balance is therefore a useful way of reducing the risk of osteoporotic fracture as you grow older.

We all have the potential to achieve excellent balance. Gymnasts, tightrope walkers, and ice skaters are shining examples of what is possible with practice. You can train yourself to have better balance by practicing flamingo swings. This balance exercise can enhance your control and flow of movement, and sharpen the reflexes that help to prevent a trip from turning into a fall. Take the opportunity to practice them whenever possible, perhaps while you are waiting for the bus or talking on the telephone.

Caution

★ If you have a history of falls or persistent balance problems, use two chairs, one either side of you for support.

Balance test

Keep a record of how long you can remain standing on one leg, even if it is only a second or two, and follow your improvement week-by-week until you can hold the position for 30 seconds.

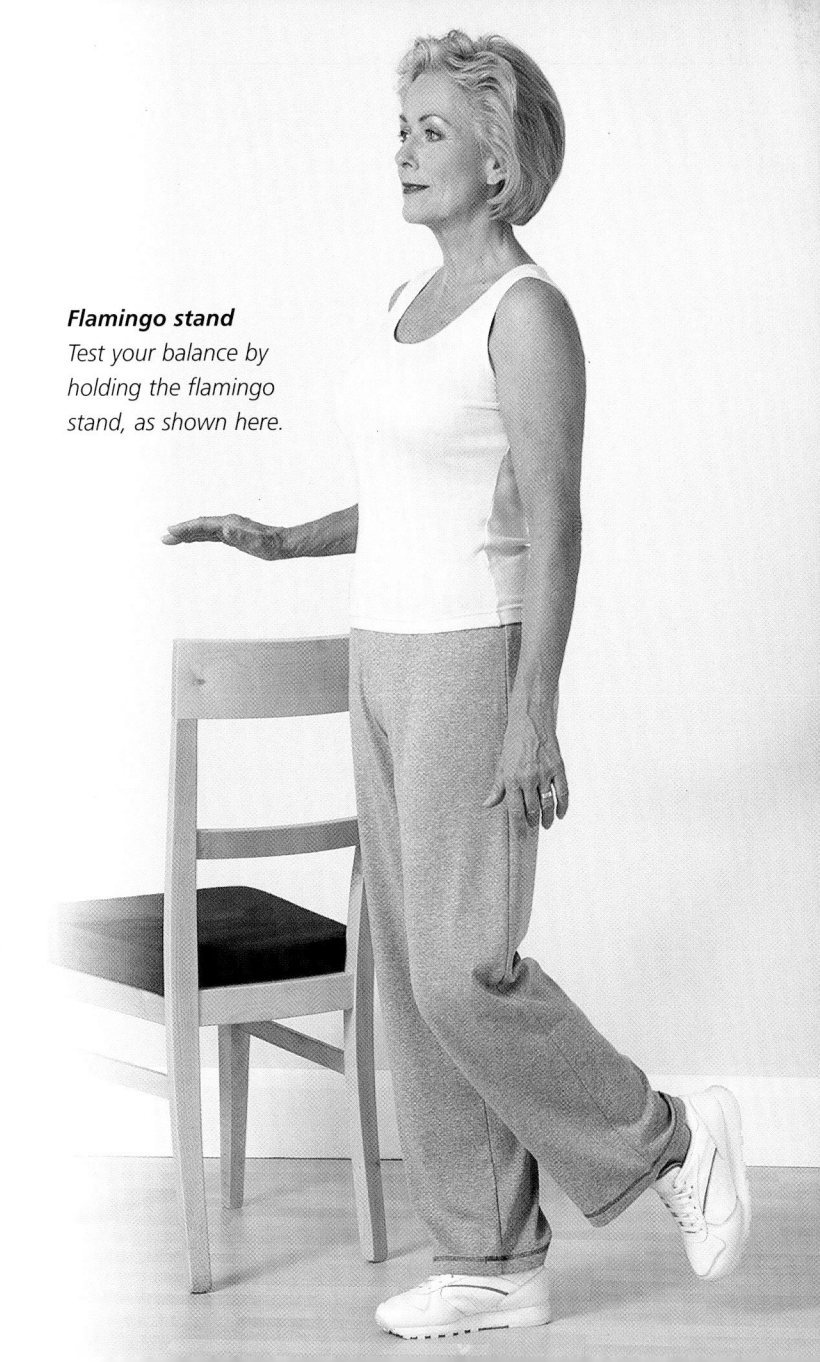

Flamingo stand
Test your balance by holding the flamingo stand, as shown here.

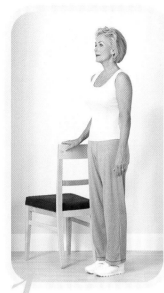

1 Stand sideways to a chair, holding the chair-back for support. Stand tall, with your feet slightly apart, and your weight distributed evenly between both feet. Relax your other arm by your side. Check your pelvic tilt and lift up out of your hips.

2 Transfer your weight onto the leg nearest to the chair. Slide your other foot forward, keeping your toes in contact with the floor. Lift the extended leg a few inches off the floor.

Look forward

Keep your chest lifted and abdominals tight

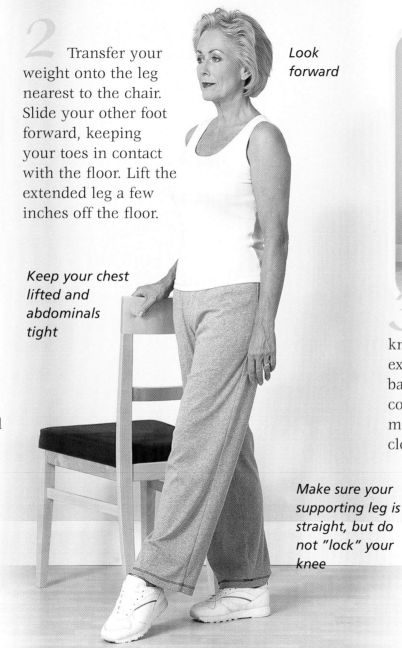

Make sure your supporting leg is straight, but do not "lock" your knee

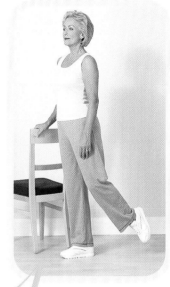

3 Keeping both knees soft, swing the extended leg gently backward in a controlled sweeping motion, keeping it close to your body.

4 Keep both hips facing forward as you swing your leg forward. Do not allow your back to arch. Repeat 6 times. Turn and repeat on the other leg.

Tandem stand & walks

Y our feet form a very small base upon which to balance your body. Successful balance requires a continuous flow of signals through the nervous system from all over the body, from the soles of your feet, eyes, middle ear, muscles, and joints.

In a Tandem Stand or Tandem Walk, the feet are placed in line, toe to heel, instead of side by side. Standing and walking on a narrower base than usual challenges the body to "fine tune" its response system.

Progression

Test your balance with a Tandem Stand. Once you can hold the position securely for ten seconds beside a wall, with both right and left leg forward, progress to the Tandem Walk exercise to improve your balance.

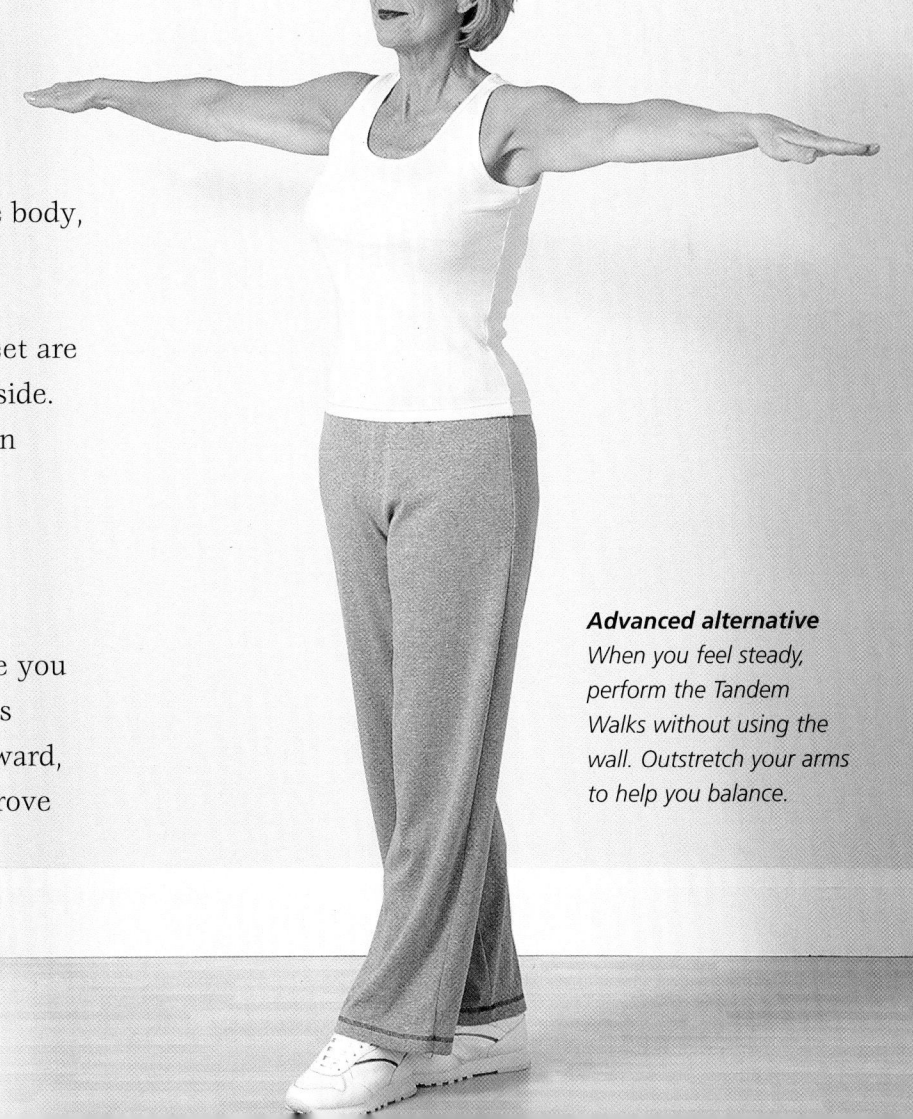

Advanced alternative
When you feel steady, perform the Tandem Walks without using the wall. Outstretch your arms to help you balance.

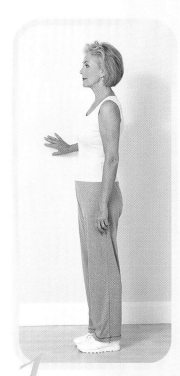

1 Tandem stand

Stand sideways to a wall and place one hand on the wall for support. Relax your other arm by your side. Stand tall, check your pelvic tilt, and tighten your abdominals.

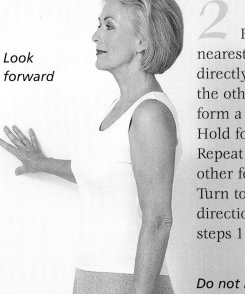

Look forward

2 Place the foot nearest the wall directly in front of the other so your feet form a straight line. Hold for 10 seconds. Repeat with your other foot in front. Turn to face the other direction and repeat steps 1 and 2.

Do not lean against the wall

Avoid rocking back on to your heels

1 Tandem walk

Use a wall for support. Place one foot directly in front of the other so your feet form a straight line. Develop this movement into continuous walking. Take 10 steps, turn slowly, and repeat in the other direction.

Caution

★ Take care not to let your back toe catch on the heel in front. Avoid turning too quickly, and take small steps to turn around.

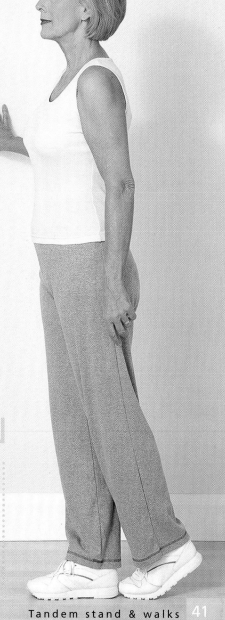

Toe walks

Purpose

This exercise improves your balance when moving. It is also good for improving calf strength and ankle flexibility.

Caution

★ If you feel unsteady, lower your heels to the floor. Rest, then begin again.

★ If you have bunions, or other foot problems that make this exercise difficult just practice Step 2, lifting your heels as much as you can. Use a chair in front for support.

These Toe Walks in combination with the Flamingo Swings and Tandem Walks provide comprehensive balance training and, if practiced regularly, will reduce your risk of falls.

When you decide to get up and walk across the room, all the right messages go to all the right muscles in just the right order. As you grow older, however, small changes to the nervous system begin to make the challenge of maintaining effective postural control more difficult, eyesight becomes less sharp and coordination slows a little. It is, therefore, increasingly important that you practice good balance as you grow older.

Progression

When you feel secure enough, you can train your balance further by doing this exercise without using a wall for support. Put your hands on your hips to start with, then raise your hands above your head for a further challenge.

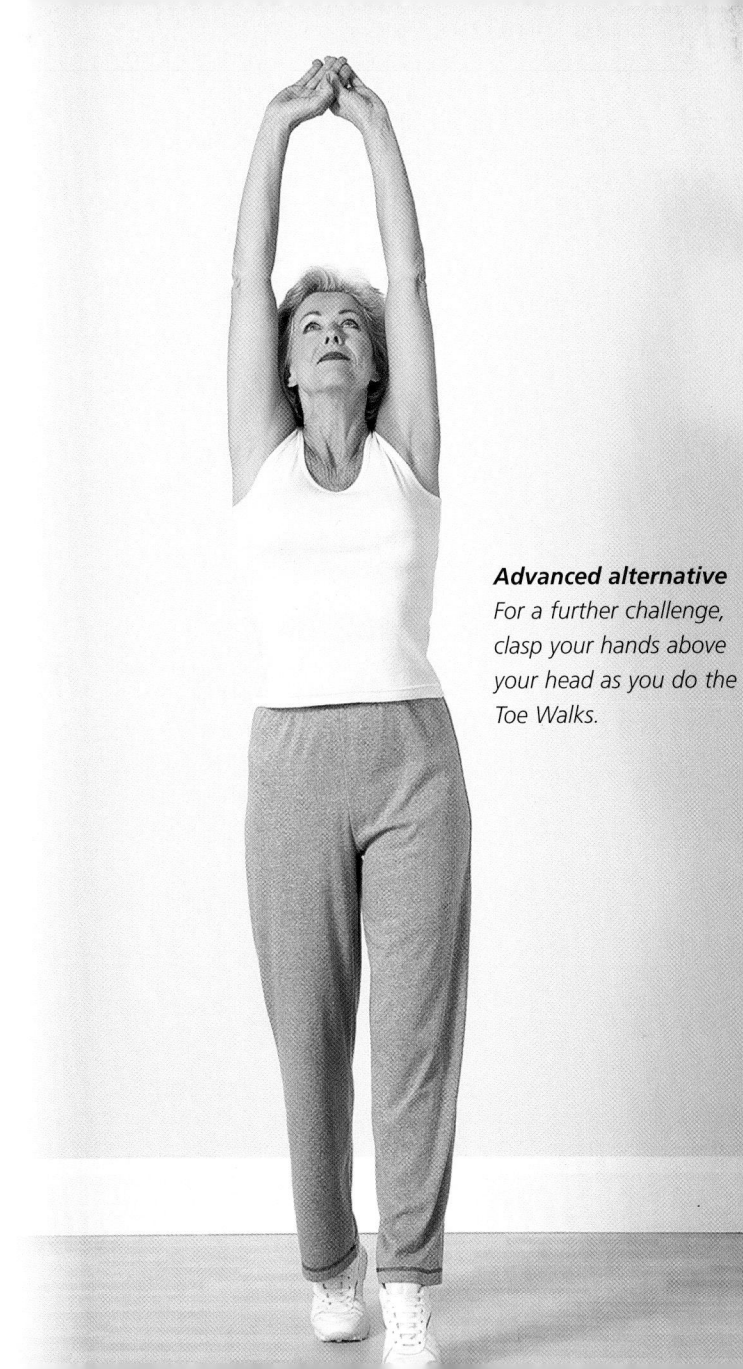

Advanced alternative
For a further challenge, clasp your hands above your head as you do the Toe Walks.

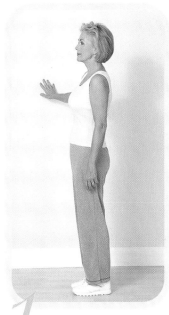

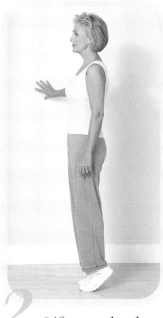

1 Stand sideways to a wall, and place one hand on the wall for support. Relax your other arm by your side. Stand tall and check your pelvic tilt.

2 Lift your heels and transfer your body weight on to the balls of your feet.

3 Using the wall as support, walk 10 steps on your toes. Then bring both feet together by stepping your back foot in. Lower your heels to the ground and turn around. Rise onto your toes and walk 10 steps in the other direction. Turn and repeat.

Keep your abdominals tight and your weight distributed evenly over both feet

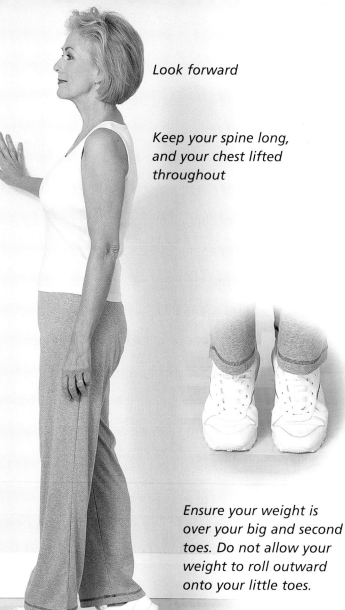

Look forward

Keep your spine long, and your chest lifted throughout

Ensure your weight is over your big and second toes. Do not allow your weight to roll outward onto your little toes.

Back lift

This exercise targets the muscles running the length of the spine (erector spinae). As their name suggests, these muscles enable you to stand erect by supporting the length of the spine.

A sedentary lifestyle does not provide sufficient action for back muscles. They are rarely exerted strongly or often enough to maintain optimum strength, so unexpected demands can cause trouble. When inadequate strength meets too large a force, damage occurs to ligaments and tendons, and the consequence is back pain. This is such a common problem that almost everyone has suffered from it at some time. Lifting a lively child or moving a heavy object can damage your back if it is not strong enough. If you have a history of back pain consult your doctor before starting and begin with the arm supported alternative below.

Progression

Begin by lifting two inches, and progress to four. Add a small flat weight across your shoulders for a further challenge. (The safety limit is 15 lbs.)

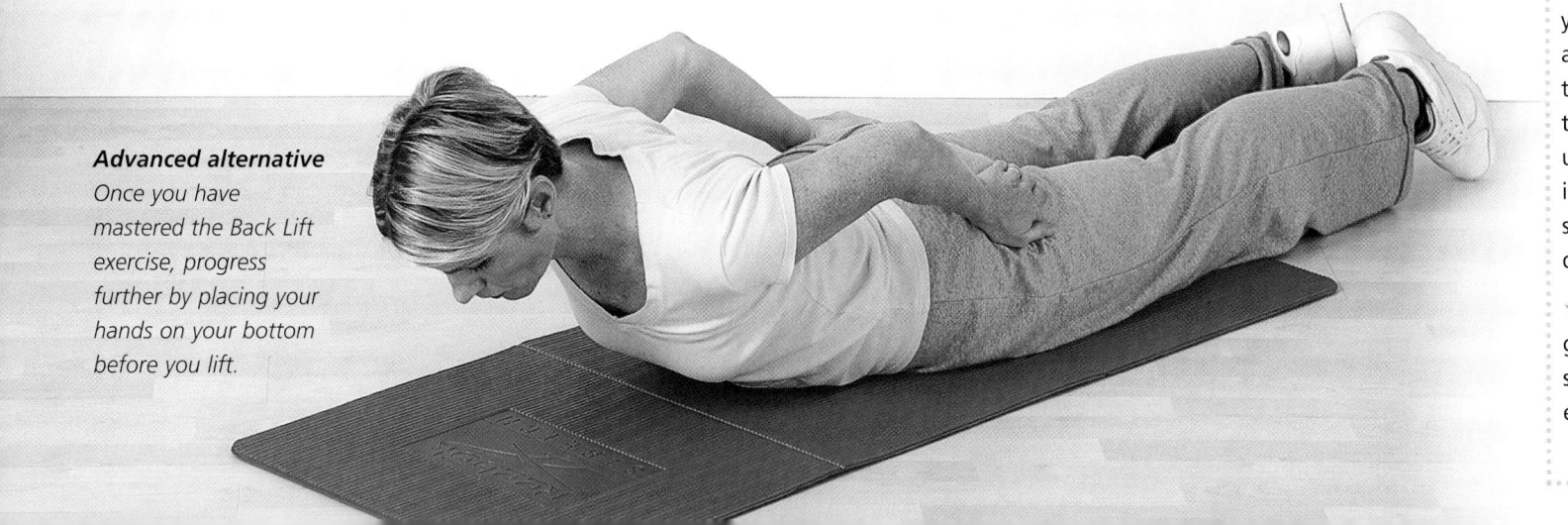

Advanced alternative
Once you have mastered the Back Lift exercise, progress further by placing your hands on your bottom before you lift.

1 Lie face-down on the floor, your legs together, your arms by your side, and your palms on the floor. Check your pelvic tilt.

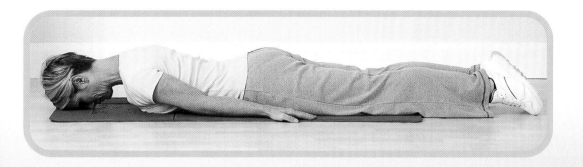

Keep the back of your neck long and your eyes looking down

Make sure your feet stay on the floor

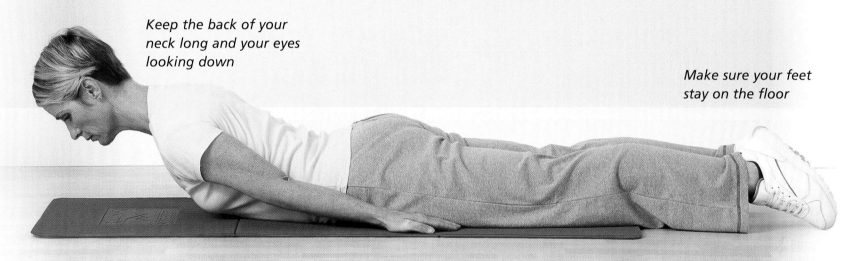

2 Lengthen your spine and lift your shoulders, back, and head off the floor. Moving slowly and with control, count to 5 to lift, hold, count to 5 to lower. Rest for 5 before repeating. Lift your palms an inch off the floor for extra challenge.

Adaptations

Start by placing your hands, palms down, under your forehead, with your elbows bent comfortably to either side. Lift and lower as for the main exercise.

Progress by placing your hands, palms down, in front of you, with your elbows under your shoulders "like a lion." Lift and lower as before.

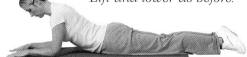

Flying **back** lift

This exercise targets many muscles especially those running the length of the spine. It is a progression of the Back Lift (see page 44) and Leg Lift (see page 48), and you should do it only when you are comfortable with the Back Lift. It will improve your shoulder flexibility and strengthen the muscles that protect your shoulder joints. This helps to prevent "frozen shoulder"; a painful condition that is common in older women. It also creates a satisfying sense of top-to-toe body line and improves body awareness and postural control.

Progression

When you have mastered the Flying Back Lift, progress by lifting your arm and leg higher to a maximum of four inches.

Advanced alternative Progress further by taking both your arms in a slow, controlled arc movement. As for the Back Lift, count to five while you complete the arc movement.

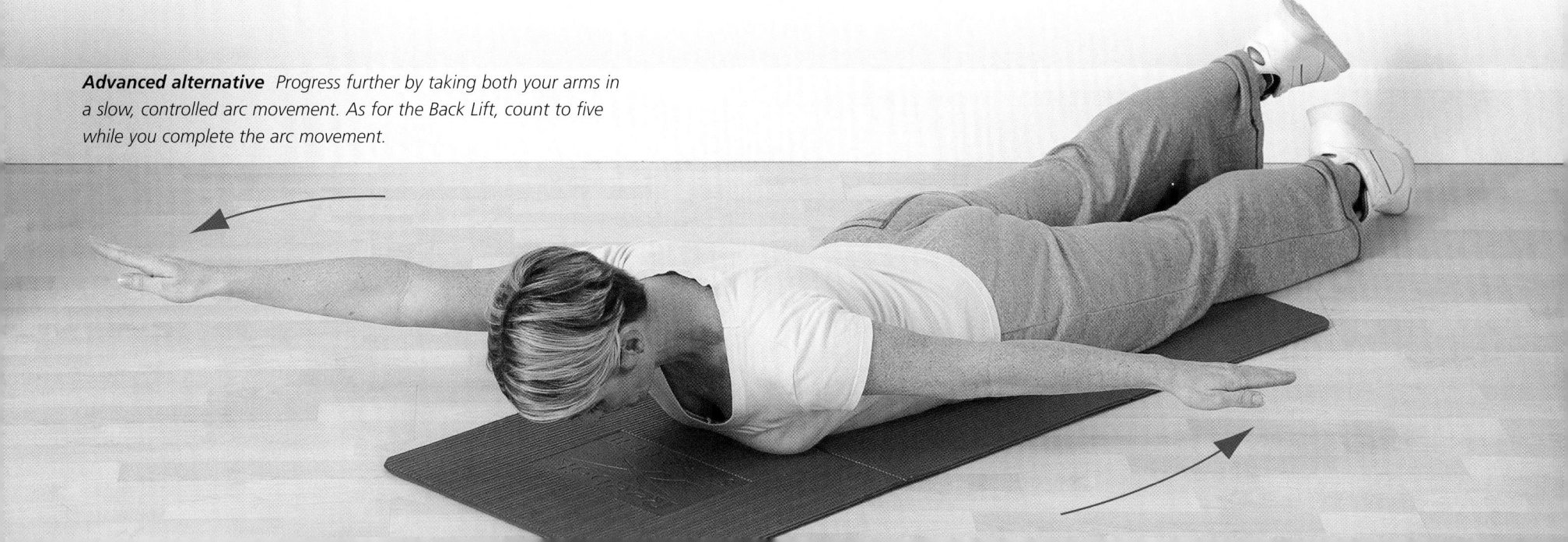

1 Lie face-down with your forehead on your folded hands. Check your pelvic tilt and tighten your abdominals.

2 Slide one palm forward along the ground. Lengthen your opposite leg along the floor away from your body.

3 Tighten your buttock muscles on this side, then lift your leg 2 inches off the floor. Maintain this position as you lengthen and lift your outstretched arm 1 inch. Count to 5 to lift, hold, and count to 5 to lower. Rest, then repeat on the other side.

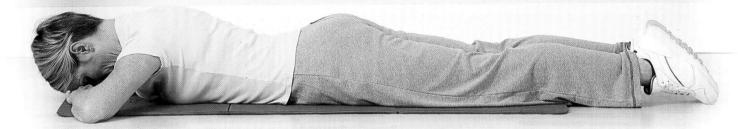

Keep the back of your neck long, your chin in, and your shoulders down throughout

Avoid over-arching your back; keep looking at the floor

Lengthen your leg as you lift

Keep your non-active foot in contact with the floor

Leg lift

This exercise targets the lower back, buttocks, and the back of the thighs (hamstrings). As you lift your leg, the muscles contract and pull on the bones of your spine and hip, which has a stimulating effect on BMD. It is also an excellent exercise for improving lower back strength, increasing the support for your lower spine, and reducing the risk of lower back pain. It will also firm up the muscles of your bottom to give you a trimmer figure. These muscles are used in all weight-bearing activities but are only challenged to their full potential during vigorous activities such as uphill running or climbing up stairs quickly.

Progression

When you have mastered the Leg Lift exercise, increase the challenge by using ankle weights.

An active life As you lift a child you use a wide range of muscles, including those in your lower back. Keeping strong will enable you to lead an active life, while minimizing risk of injury.

1 Lie face-down with your legs together and your forehead on your folded hands. Check your pelvic tilt, and tighten your abdominals.

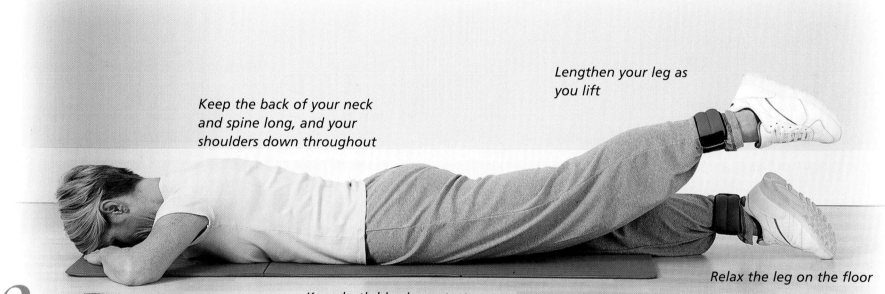

Keep the back of your neck and spine long, and your shoulders down throughout

Lengthen your leg as you lift

Relax the leg on the floor

Keep both hips in contact with the floor

2 Lengthen one leg backward along the floor, tighten your buttock muscles on this side, and keeping both hips pressed into the floor, lift your leg a few inches. Lengthen and lift another inch upward, then lower. Count to 3 to lift, hold, count to 3 to lower. Rest, then repeat on the other side.

Common mistake

★ Do not lift your leg so high that your hip lifts off the floor. This can place strain on your back.

Side leg lift

This exercise targets the large outer thigh muscles (the abductors), which are attached across the top of the femur to the outer edges of the pelvic girdle. These muscles are used when you step sideways but are rarely used to their full potential. If you make them work against some resistance, the underlying bone is stimulated.

Progression

Start without weights and with bent knees. Add a light weight around your thigh to progress, and then move the weight to your ankle to further increase the resistance.

Purpose

To increase bone mineral density (BMD) in the hip. It also strengthens the muscles on the outside of the hip and thigh.

Caution

★ If you have an artificial hip, start and finish with your knees bent and a cushion between your thighs.

Advanced alternative *Progress further by lifting with your top leg straight.*

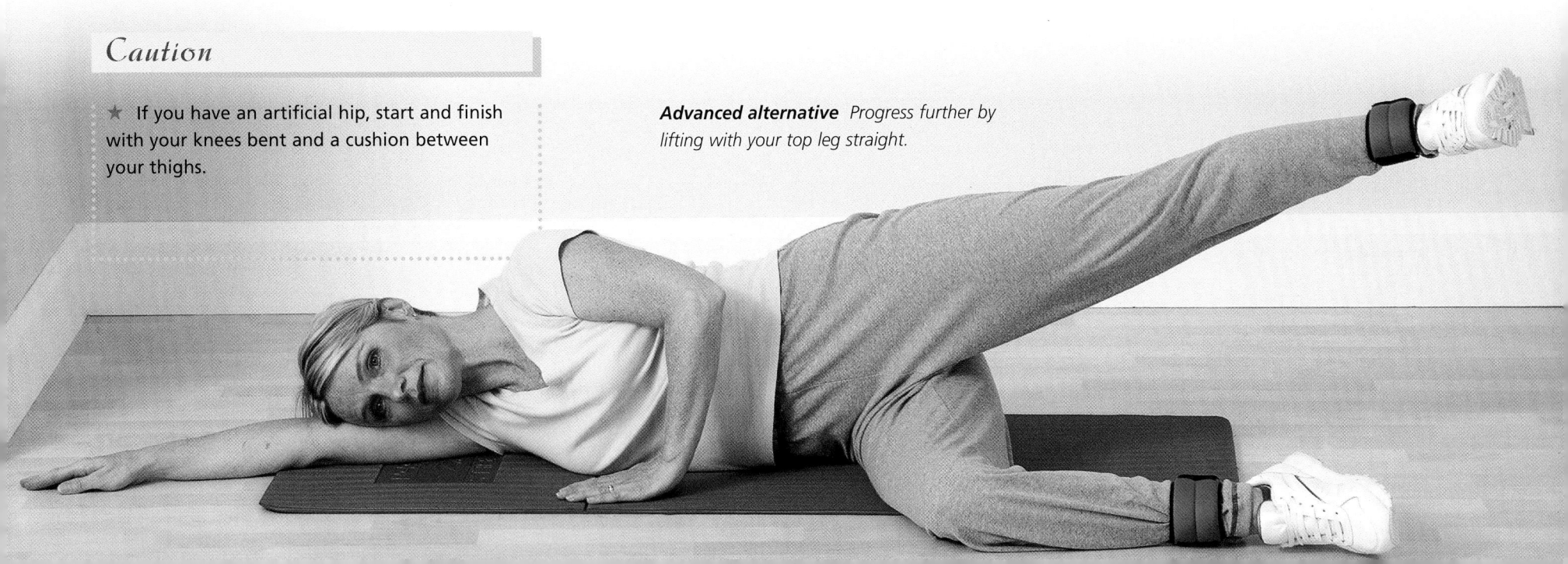

1 Lie sideways with your knees and hips at right angles, with weights around your ankles. Rest your head on your lower arm or a cushion for comfort. Place your other hand on the mat, opposite your chest. Check your pelvic tilt, and tighten your abdominals.

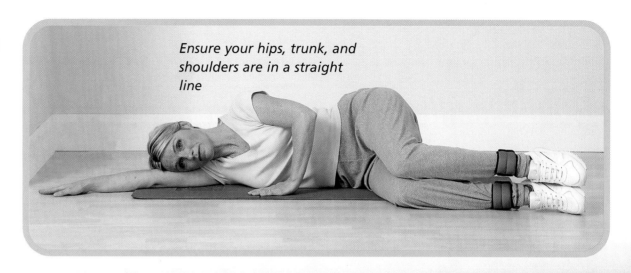

Ensure your hips, trunk, and shoulders are in a straight line

2 Taking care to keep your knee and foot facing forward and slightly down, raise your top leg about 3 inches. Count to 3 to lift, hold, count to 3 to lower. Rest, then repeat. Roll over on to your other side and repeat with your other leg.

Take care not to let your top hip and knee roll back

Keep your knee and ankle at the same height

Thigh squeeze

Caution

★ If you experience any pain in your pubic area or lower back, check your pelvic tilt, and move a little further away from your partner. If the pain persists, stop, and try doing the exercise on your own using a resistance ball.

This exercise targets the inner thigh muscles (adductors), which pull the legs together. You use these muscles when horse-riding or swimming breaststroke, but on the whole, hip adduction is an unusual activity in everyday life. Exercising these muscles provides unusual forces for the underlying skeleton to resist, which is why it helps to improve the density in the hip.

Although swimming is a healthy activity, the forces are not high enough to stimulate bone. This is because the water yields as you kick. To load your bones, you need to work against a bigger resistance. A resistance ball is ideal, but it is fun and effective if you can work with a partner. It is important to choose a partner of similar size and strength to yourself. The added advantage is that while you are exercising your adductors, your partner is exercising her abductors (the outer thigh muscles), and vice versa when you swap.

Progression

Just squeeze as hard as you can.

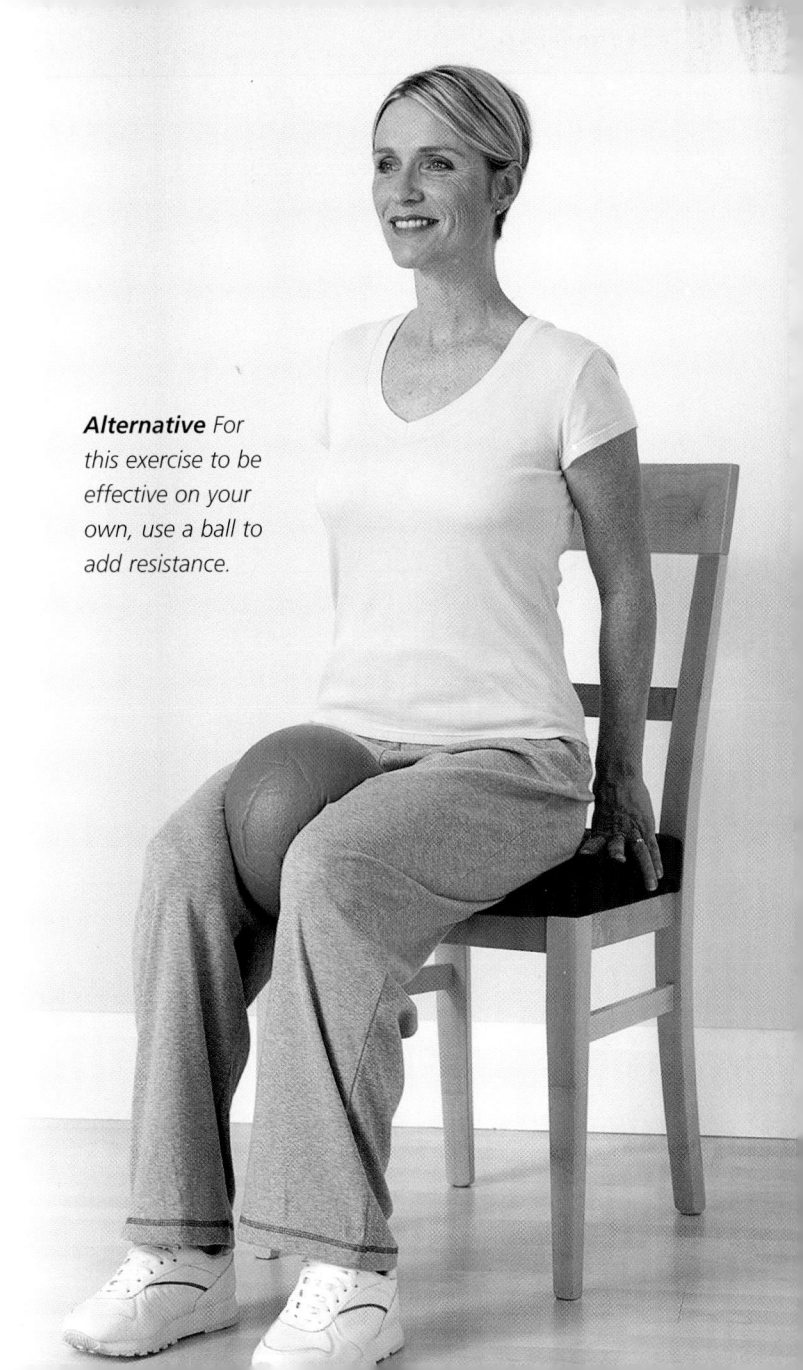

Alternative For this exercise to be effective on your own, use a ball to add resistance.

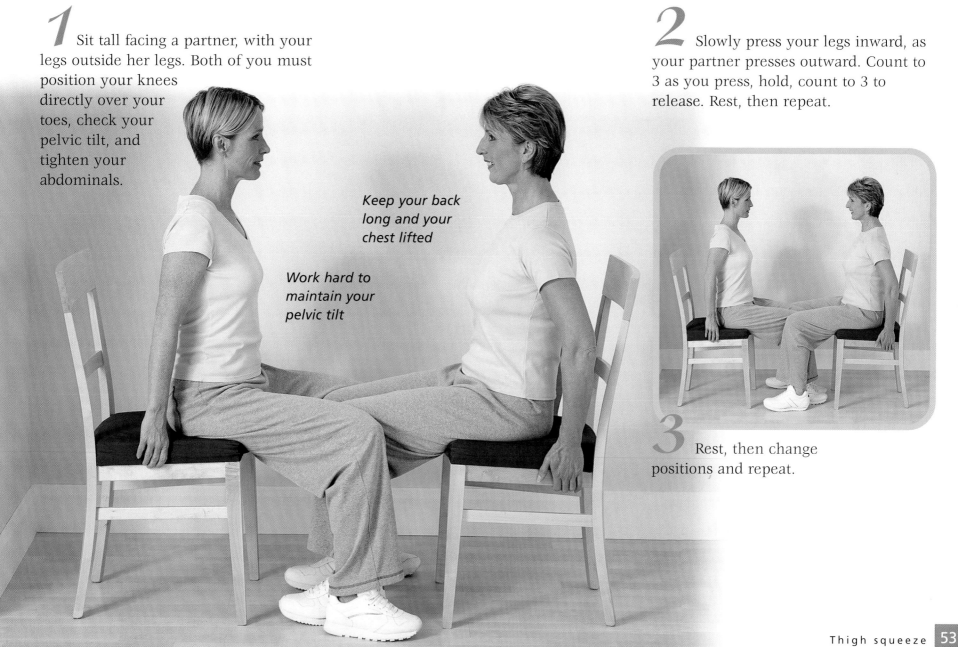

1 Sit tall facing a partner, with your legs outside her legs. Both of you must position your knees directly over your toes, check your pelvic tilt, and tighten your abdominals.

Keep your back long and your chest lifted

Work hard to maintain your pelvic tilt

2 Slowly press your legs inward, as your partner presses outward. Count to 3 as you press, hold, count to 3 to release. Rest, then repeat.

3 Rest, then change positions and repeat.

Leg press

Purpose

To load the hip bone and strengthen the muscles at the front and back of the hips, thighs, and knees.

Caution

★ If you have knee problems take care not to lock your knees.

★ If you have an artificial hip do not lift the thigh into the chest; begin with the knee at hip height.

This exercise targets the muscles that straighten the hip, including the quadriceps, so it is good for increasing BMD in these areas. You use these muscles when you push off against the floor to rise from a chair or climb stairs. Activities like jogging and jumping also challenge these muscles, and in turn, promote BMD.

It is difficult to provide enough resistance in a home exercise for this group of muscles. You need to use both arms to provide resistance for one leg; if you still find it easy to stretch out the strongest band, use a weight-training machine in a gym to provide sufficient resistance. You will be surprised at how much you can push with your legs; these muscles can resist at least five times your body weight, for example, when you are jumping (see page 88).

Progression

You can develop this exercise by using increasingly strong bands, by doubling your band, or by tying the band around the back of a chair seat rather than holding the ends.

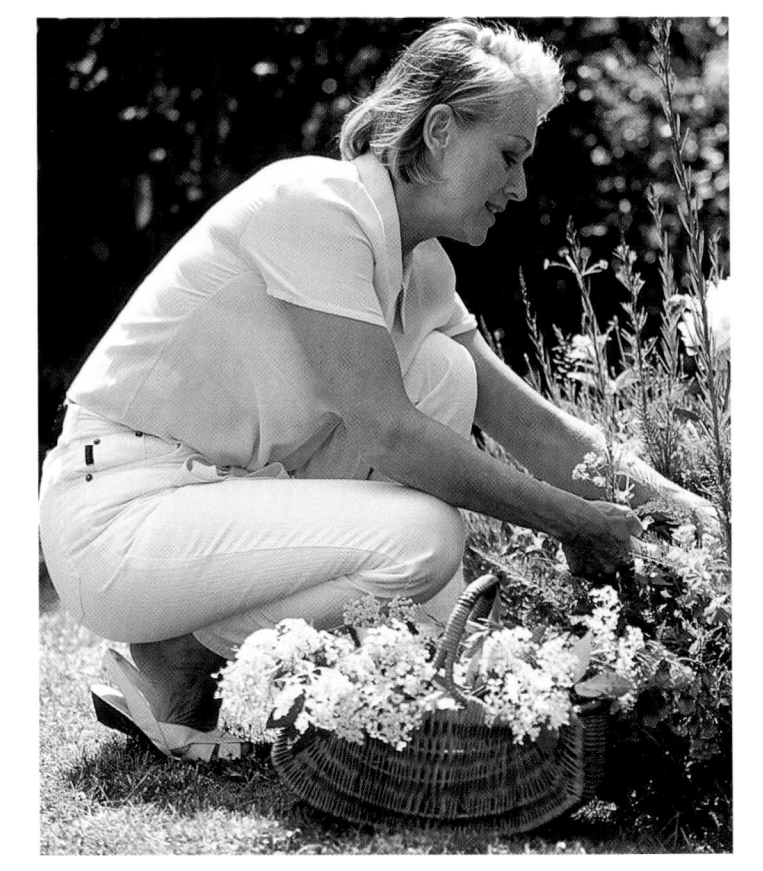

Picking flowers *There are many everyday tasks that require us to squat down on our haunches. When we stand up from this position, we use a powerful leg press.*

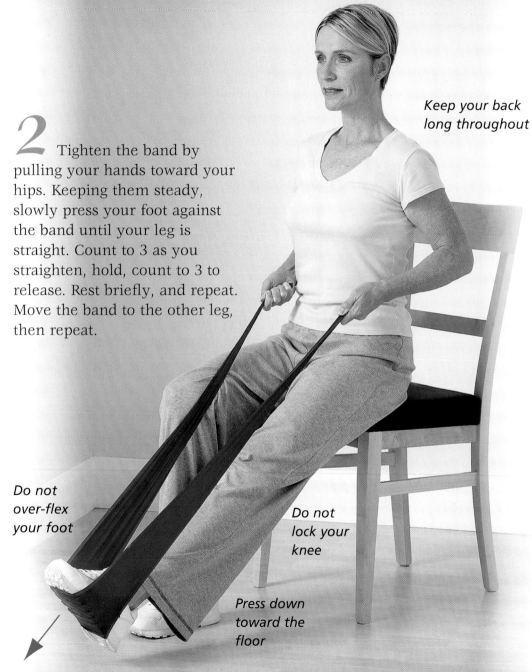

2 Tighten the band by pulling your hands toward your hips. Keeping them steady, slowly press your foot against the band until your leg is straight. Count to 3 as you straighten, hold, count to 3 to release. Rest briefly, and repeat. Move the band to the other leg, then repeat.

Keep your back long throughout

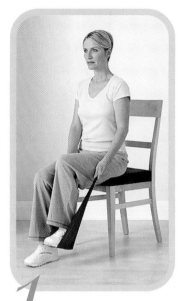

1 Sit tall with your feet and legs hip-width apart and your knees directly over your ankles. Place a resistance band under the ball of one foot and hold one end firmly in each hand. Check your pelvic tilt, tighten your abdominals, and lift your thigh toward your chest.

Do not over-flex your foot

Do not lock your knee

Press down toward the floor

Adaptation

If you find holding the band taut uncomfortable, hold it against the chair seat instead.

Common mistake

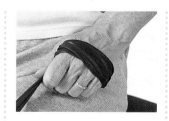

★ Do not wrap the band around your hand.

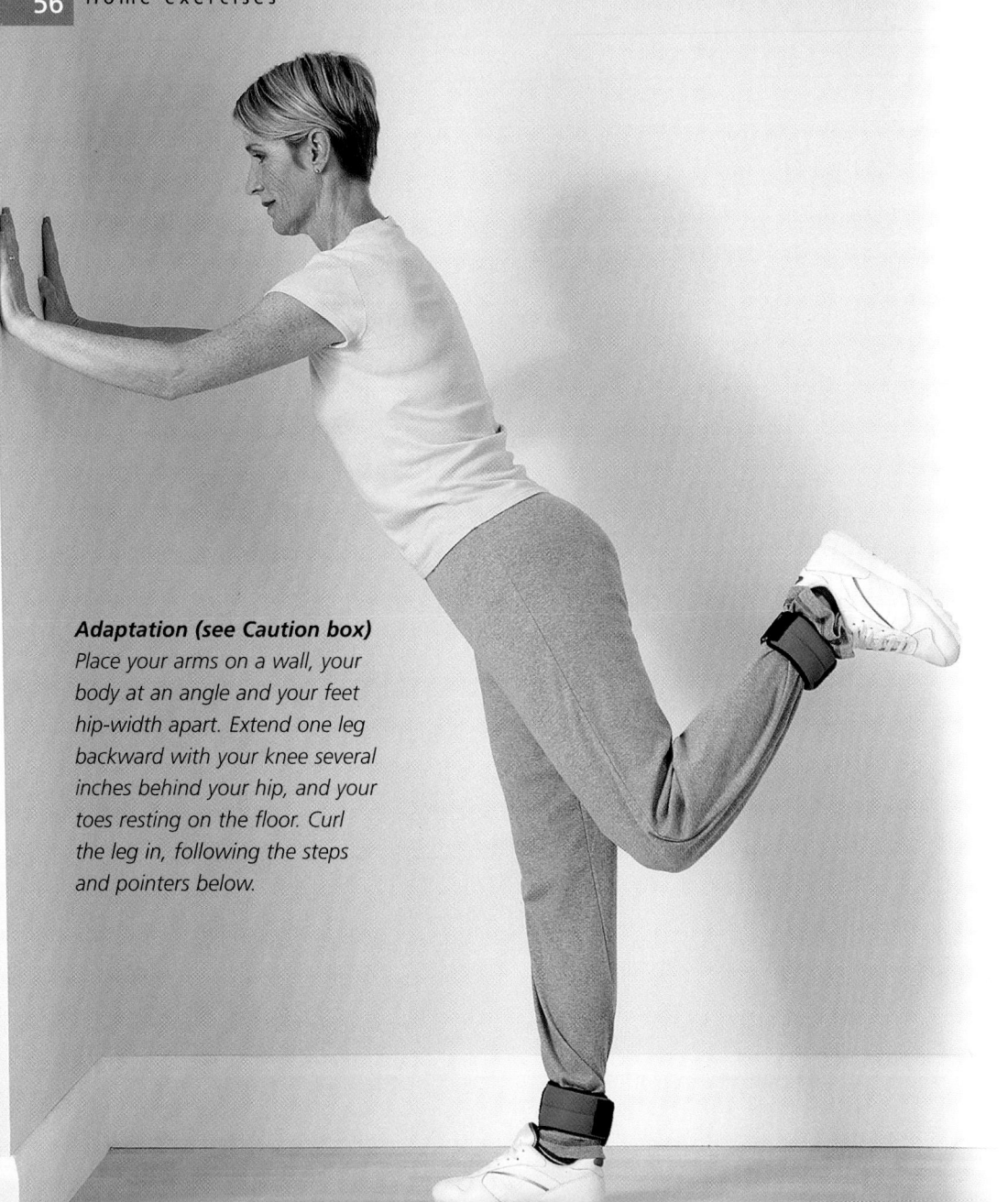

Adaptation (see Caution box)
Place your arms on a wall, your body at an angle and your feet hip-width apart. Extend one leg backward with your knee several inches behind your hip, and your toes resting on the floor. Curl the leg in, following the steps and pointers below.

Leg curl

This exercise targets the large muscles at the back of the thigh (the hamstrings) which straighten the hip and bend the knees.

The hamstrings are potentially powerful muscles but they are often weaker than they should be when compared to their opposite muscle group: the quadriceps. The hamstrings are used in everyday activities, such as stair-climbing, and for many sports, but they need extra resistance to improve strength and load the bones. The Leg Curl loads bones effectively only when you use ankle weights.

Progression

Master the exercise using a light ankle weight, then increase the weight and the height of the lift to a limit of three inches. (The safety limit is 20 lbs).

Purpose
To increase bone mineral density (BMD) at the hip and strengthen the muscles at the back of the thigh.

1 Kneel on all-fours with your legs hip-width apart. Your elbows should be bent under your shoulders, with your forearms and palms flat on the floor. Check your pelvic tilt, tighten your abdominals, and slide one leg out behind you. Flex your foot and lift it 1 inch. Lengthen your leg.

2 Continue to lift your straight leg until your knee is just above the level of your hip, then curl the lower leg inward to a count of 3 until your ankle is directly above your knee.

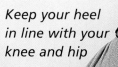

Keep your heel in line with your knee and hip

Your foot should stay flexed

Caution

★ If you feel any discomfort in your joints, neck or head, or are unable to get to the floor safely, do the standing alternative.

★ If you are postmenopausal, do the standing alternative.

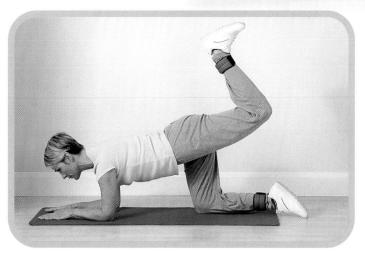

3 Taking care not to over-arch your back, lift your leg 1 inch, hold, then lower with control for a count of 3. Rest, then repeat. Repeat with the other leg.

Straight **leg** lift

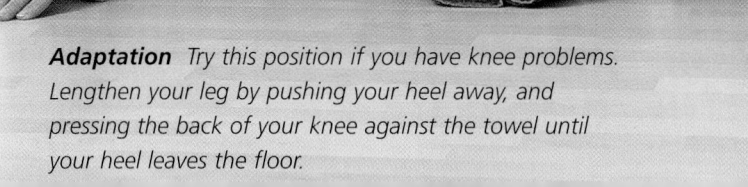

This exercise targets the quadriceps muscles of the thigh that cross both the front of the hip (the hip flexors) and the front of the knees (the knee extensors). They are powerful muscles that you use to some extent in all weight-bearing activities; it is the most important muscle for cycling or kicking. This exercise challenges the four quadricep muscles to their full potential, and loads the hip. It is also excellent for helping to reduce instability and discomfort arising from incorrect alignment of the knee joints. Keeping these muscles strong is important for independence as you grow older.

Performing this exercise in a controlled way and progressing step-by-step is very important if you are to get the maximum benefit.

Progression

Add a weight when you have mastered the Straight Leg Lift. Progress further by lifting the heel about four inches off the floor. Do not lift higher than your other thigh. Progress further by increasing the weight.

Adaptation Try this position if you have knee problems. Lengthen your leg by pushing your heel away, and pressing the back of your knee against the towel until your heel leaves the floor.

Purpose
To increase bone mineral density (BMD) in the hips, strengthen the thighs, and stabilize the knees.

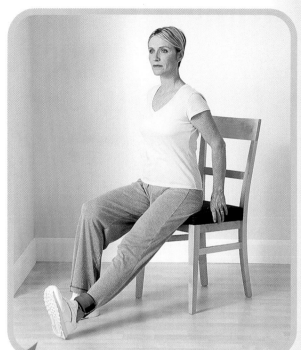

1 Sit toward the front of a chair, with your legs hip-width apart. Sit tall with your knees directly over your ankles. Hold the chair seat to support your back. Keeping your foot in contact with the floor, slowly slide one leg forward.

2 Lengthen your leg as much as possible by pushing your heel away, then check your pelvic tilt and tighten your abdominals and thigh muscles. Count to 3 as you lift your foot slowly, 1–2 inches, hold, then lower it with control for 3. Rest, then repeat with the other leg.

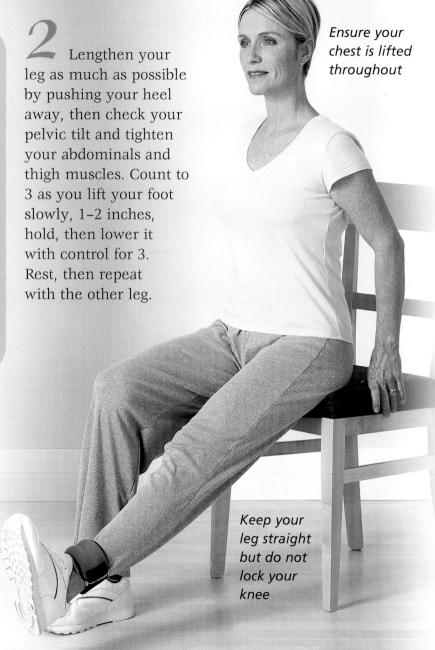

Ensure your chest is lifted throughout

Keep your leg straight but do not lock your knee

Caution

★ If you feel any pain or discomfort in your back or knees during this exercise, check your pelvic tilt, abdominals, and leg alignment. If the problem persists, discontinue this exercise, and seek advice from your doctor.

★ Avoid the temptation to lift too high or use ankle weights too soon.

Thigh lift

Caution

★ If you feel any pain in your back, hip, or knees, other than mild stiffness following this exercise, try it without weights. If the pain persists, seek advice from your doctor.

★ Do not lift your leg higher than shown.

This exercise targets several muscles that bend the hip joint, but the important one for bone loading is the psoas muscle which crosses from the femur to the lumbar spine. This exercise has been shown to be effective on its own, rather than as part of a package; it is usual to evaluate at least six weight-training exercises together. Performed at least three times a week using a 10 lb weight on the mid-thigh, this exercise has been shown to maintain BMD in postmenopausal women.

You use these muscles a little when you lift your foot to step onto a bus and a lot when you lean backward if sitting without a support.

Progression

Master the exercise using just the weight of your leg, then add a light weight around your thigh as shown and lift just one inch. Progress by lifting another inch or two without letting your chest or lower back sag. Progress further by moving the weight further down your thigh toward your knee, then increase the weight.

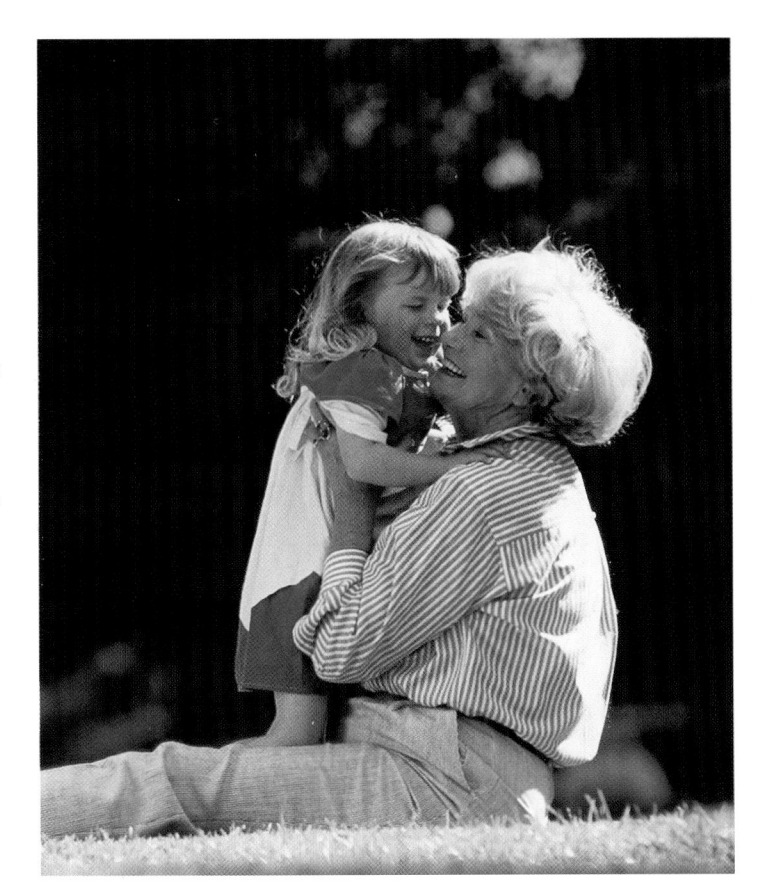

Active living Even simple, everyday activities require strength; the woman in this position requires strong hip and thigh muscles to resist the weight of the child and her own upper body.

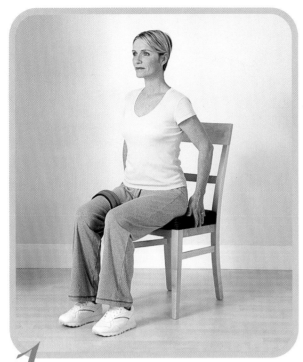

1 Sit toward the front of a chair with your feet hip-width apart and your knees directly over your ankles. Secure a weight across the top of one thigh. Sit tall and hold the chair to support your back. Check your pelvic tilt and tighten your abdominals.

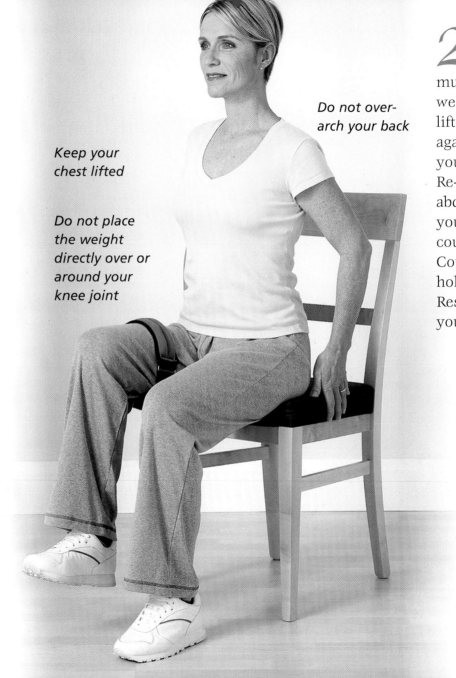

Do not over-arch your back

Keep your chest lifted

Do not place the weight directly over or around your knee joint

2 Tense the muscles of your weighted thigh as if to lift the leg. Press down against the floor with your supporting foot. Re-tighten your abdominals and lift your weighted thigh a couple of inches. Count to 3 as you lift, hold, count to 3 lower. Rest, then repeat with your other leg.

Wrist curl

Caution

★ If you experience pain at the end of the upward or downward movement you have gone beyond your natural range.

Most women have weak arms compared to their legs, so it is well worth doing some upper body exercises. The wrist is particularly vulnerable to osteoporotic fracture, so the next few exercises concentrate on increasing wrist BMD. The wrist curl targets the muscles which cross the wrist. To identify these muscles, hold your forearm gently in one hand while you clench your other hand into a fist; you will feel your muscles contracting. The muscles provide your grip power for twisting the lids off jars.

The wrist is an extremely flexible joint which allows the hand to move in all three planes like a swivel arm desk lamp. The forearm muscles pull on the wrist bones as you lift the weight, and the force is greater while you lower the weight because the muscles control the pull of gravity.

Progression

Master the Wrist Curl exercise using a light weight, and progress further by increasing the weight. (The safety limit is 12 lbs in each hand.)

Loading the wrist bones *Hammering like this uses a wrist curl action with the wrist in a different position; the impact will probably help to load the wrist bones.*

Alternative

Both exercises can be performed double-handed provided you can find a suitable surface, such as a waist-height narrow table or bench, where your back can be erect and your forearms supported.

1 Sit toward the front of a chair with your feet hip-width apart and your knees over your ankles. Hold a dumbbell in an underhand grip, with your wrist horizontal and in line with your elbow. Support your forearm with your other hand, resting it on your thigh. Lean forward slightly.

Ensure your back is long and your chest lifted

Keep your shoulders facing forward

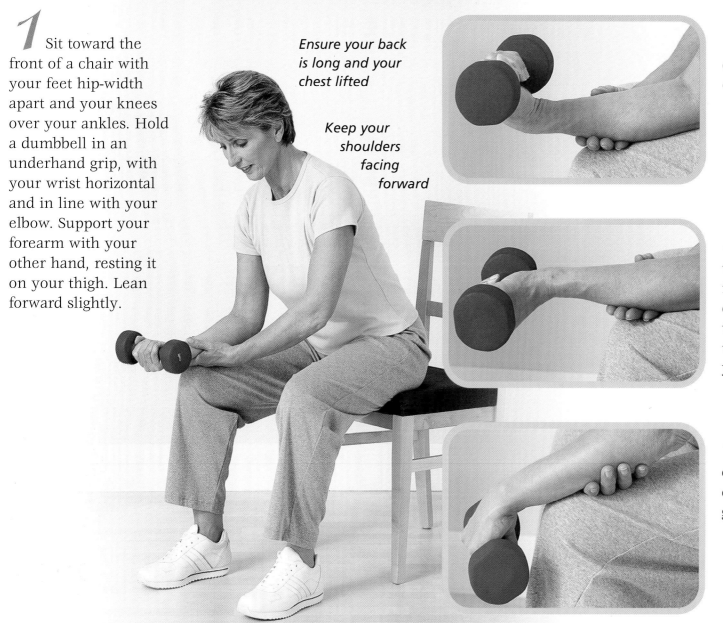

2 Count to 3 to curl the dumbbell upward, moving only your wrist. Hold.

3 Count to 3 to lower the weight until your wrist is fully extended downward, and return it the start position. Rest, then repeat. Repeat with your other arm.

4 Turn your forearm over and repeat the exercise using an overhand grip.

Arm curl

This exercise, often referred to as a biceps curl, targets the biceps muscle at the front of your upper arm—the muscle that everyone pinches to see if you are strong. It is attached to the radius and the humerus bones.

The exercise uses the biceps muscles to bend the elbow joints, and then allows them to straighten again resisting the force of gravity acting on the hand-held weights. These curls will make your biceps feel firm, and give your arm a good line without becoming bulgy. You'll find it easier to manage heavy shopping bags as your muscles increase in strength. This exercise will help to improve BMD in the wrists, because they are also involved in the lift.

Progression

If you find this exercise hard, then try with one arm at a time. Master the technique with a light weight, then progress by increasing the weight. (The safety limit is 20 lbs in each hand.)

Controlled movement Curl your arms slowly, and with control, for a satisfying and effective exercise.

1 Stand tall with your feet hip-width apart and your knees bent slightly. Your arms should be a little more than shoulder-width apart. Hold the dumbbells in an underhand grip with your palms facing forward. Check your pelvic tilt, tighten your abdominals, press your shoulders back and down, and lengthen your arms.

Keep your elbows and knees soft

2 Curl your arms upward toward your shoulders. Count to 3 as you lift, hold, and count to 3 to lower. Rest, then repeat.

Make sure that your wrists stay straight

Hold your upper body still

Keep your abdominals tight

Distribute your weight evenly between both feet, and think tall

Common mistake

★ Do not lean back as you lift your arms or swing the weight upward. Think of keeping the body firm and still as you lift and lower.

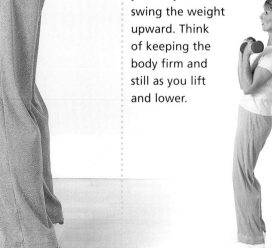

Arm press

Purpose

To increase the bone mineral density (BMD) in your wrists and to strengthen the muscles at the back of your arms, and in your back.

Caution

★ If you have a shoulder injury, place your hands below shoulder height.

★ If you have arthritis in your fingers, shoulders, or neck, do not perform the alternative opposite.

This exercise targets the muscles across the chest and upper arm (pectorals) and at the back of your upper arm (triceps); it also involves your wrist muscles, particularly when the "spring" is added to the press (see Progression). It is a vertical press-up, which is much easier to perform than a horizontal one. As well as being good for your wrist BMD, it helps you to maintain your upper body muscles and a good bust line. The triceps area, in particular, can become "baggy" as you get older, if neglected.

You need to hold your body firm in this exercise, which requires concentration. Think of your body as a rigid plank of wood, with your arms doing all the work.

Progression

You can add impact by performing the spring alternative shown right. Push away a little more powerfully until your hands leave the wall, and then land carefully, rolling your weight through your fingers, palm, and heel of your hand.

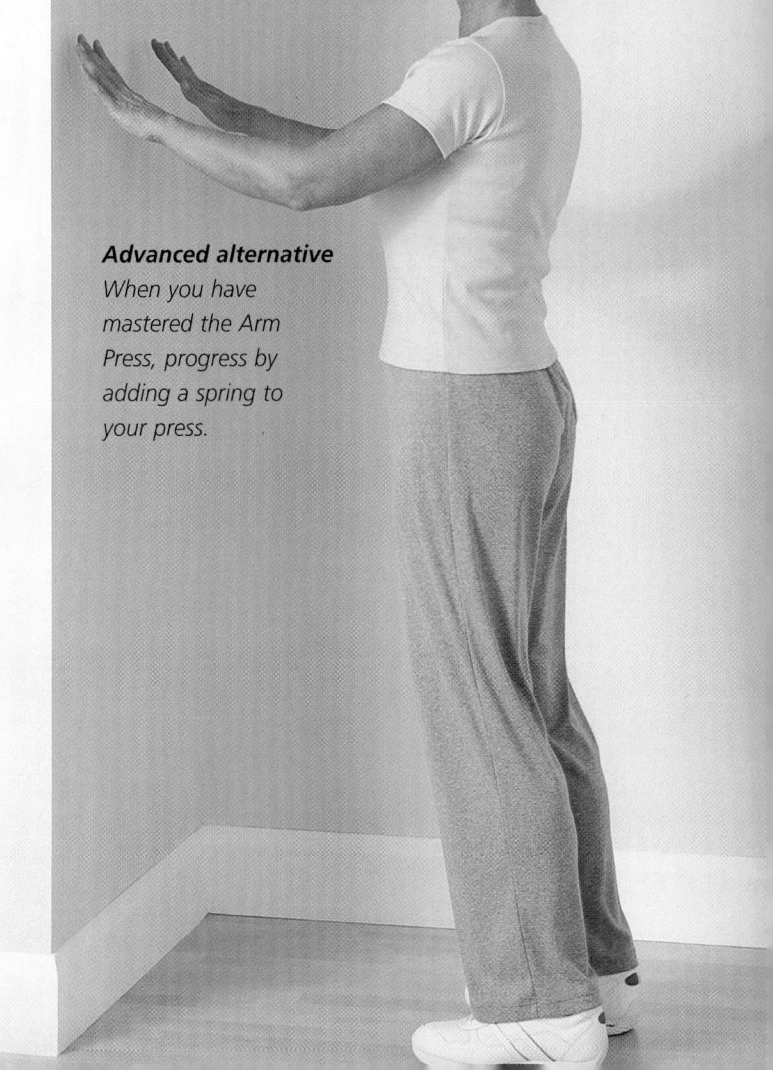

Advanced alternative
When you have mastered the Arm Press, progress by adding a spring to your press.

1 Stand facing a wall with your feet hip-width apart. Place your palms, fingers upward, on the wall at shoulder height. Your arms should be shoulder-width apart, and your elbows extended but not locked. Check your pelvic tilt and tighten your abdominals.

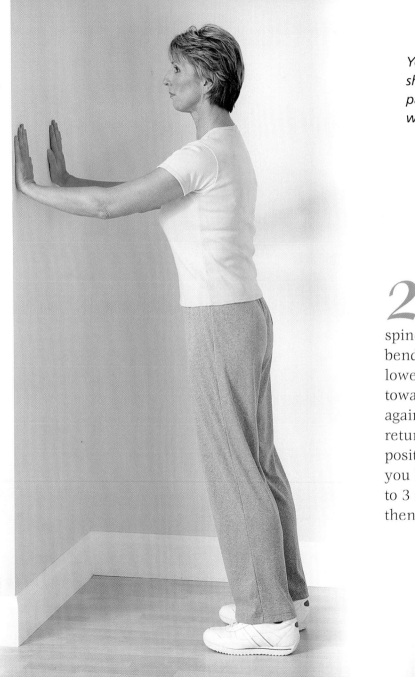

Your forehead should be parallel to the wall

Keep your shoulders down

Do not over-arch your back

2 Keeping your spine and neck long, bend your elbows and lower your body toward the wall. Press against the wall to return to your start position. Count to 3 as you lower, hold, count to 3 to return. Rest, then repeat.

Keep your heels on the floor

Shoulder press

This exercise targets the muscles across the top of the shoulder joint and the triceps at the back of the arm; it requires a good range of movement in the shoulder. You use these muscles when you lift something onto a high shelf. The exercise also involves your pectoral muscles and the muscles of the upper back and spine, so it should help improve BMD in the spine. The spine has to be like a firm pole to keep the weight of the arms and the dumbbells in position. If you do not observe the caution box (left), the risk of shoulder injury is high.

Progression

Start cautiously with a light weight and increase gradually as you become more competent (the safety limit is 15 lbs in each hand). For variety, turn your forearms and palms inward to perform the press. The seated version helps to stabilize the lower back and is therefore safer when using heavier weights. Do not perform the standing alternative unless you are very competent.

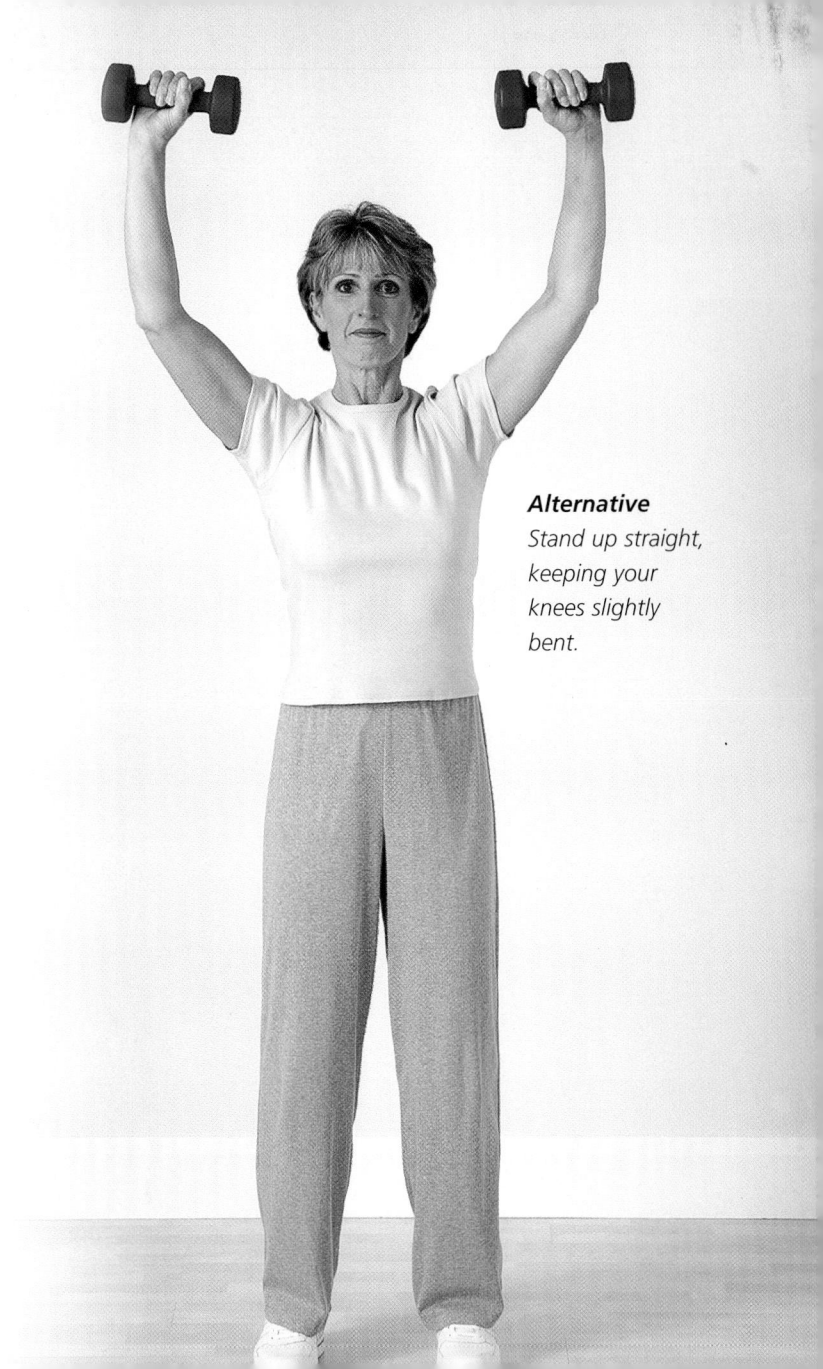

Alternative
Stand up straight, keeping your knees slightly bent.

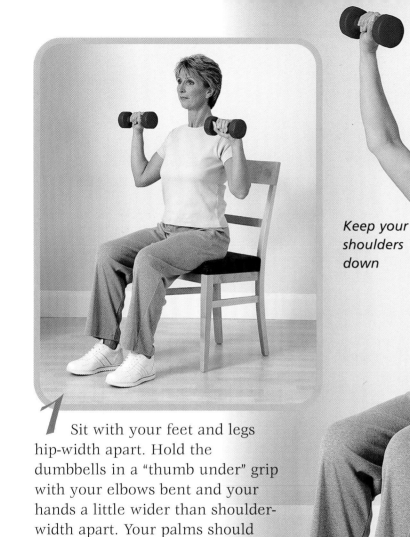

Push directly upward

★ Don't push your arms forward: this places strain on your back.

★ Don't allow your arms to swing as you lift or lower.

Do not lock your elbows

Keep your shoulders down

Avoid over-arching your back

1 Sit with your feet and legs hip-width apart. Hold the dumbbells in a "thumb under" grip with your elbows bent and your hands a little wider than shoulder-width apart. Your palms should face forward with your knuckles up toward the ceiling. Check your pelvic tilt and tighten your abdominals.

2 Press the dumbbells directly up until your arms are as straight as possible but not locked. Count to 3 as you lift, hold, count to 3 as you lower to the start position. Rest, then repeat.

Chest press

This exercise targets the muscles that straighten the forearm and many supporting muscles in the back and chest, including the pectorals. You use these muscles to push heavy objects around, for example, when you re-arrange the furniture or give children a push on the swing. This exercise will firm up your bust-line, as well as helping to improve BMD in the spine.

The arm action is similar to that in the Shoulder Press but the forces are acting in a different direction so the loading on the spine will be different. It is less demanding of the supporting muscles and is feasible even if you have a poor range of movement in the shoulder.

Progression

Increase the weights to work your muscles harder. (The safety limit is 20 lbs in each hand.) This floor chest press effectively loads the wrists and spine. Benefits to the spine are greater if you go to a gym and use a chest press machine.

Purpose

To increase BMD in your wrists and spine and strengthen the muscles of your chest, shoulders, and back.

Caution

★ Attention to the position of the weight is particularly important for safety in this exercise.

★ If you experience dizziness when you get up from the floor, make sure you come up slowly.

Alternative This exercise can be performed just as effectively with a body bar instead of the dumbbells.

1 Lie on a mat with your knees bent, your feet and legs hip-width apart, and your feet on the floor. Hold the dumbbells in an overhand grip, your palms facing forward, and your knuckles facing the ceiling. Your arms should be bent and slightly wider than shoulder-width apart. Check your pelvic tilt, and tighten your abdominals. Press the dumbbells upward, without locking the elbows to reach the start position.

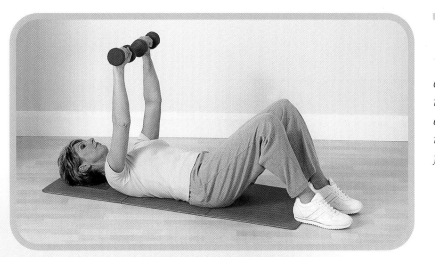

Alternative

You can do an effective chest press while seated by using a band instead of dumbbells if you are unable to get to the floor safely.

Keep the dumbbells in line with your chest, not your neck

2 Slowly lower the dumbbells to a count of 3 by bending your elbows, allowing your arms to move out to the sides until they touch the floor. Rest, but maintain the arm and wrist position. Press the dumbbells up again to a count of 3. Hold in the start position, then repeat.

Avoid over-arching or flattening your back

All-fours

Purpose

To increase bone mineral density (BMD) in the wrists and strengthen the muscles of the wrists, forearms, and shoulders.

This exercise is a weight-bearing exercise for your arms rather than your legs. It targets many of the same muscles as the Arm Press (see page 66), particularly the pectorals, triceps, and wrist flexors. The loading on your wrist, however, is greater than in an arm press. When you are on all-fours, your forearms are carrying nearly half of your body weight. By moving the position of your hands on the floor you can vary the direction of loading and the way that your wrist muscles are pulling to support your weight.

This exercise, along with the Arm Press and the Wrist Press, Twist, & Pull (see page 74), forms a set of bone-loading exercises, which load the wrist in different directions. Research has shown that, when all these exercises were done three times a week by postmenopausal women, they improved BMD in the wrists by almost six percent.

You load your wrist in a similar way when you polish a table, clean the windows, or push a child along in a stroller. Pushing a stroller probably achieves just as much as this set of exercises, provided the child weighs over 20 lbs. Going uphill with a stroller provides a wrist press, downhill a wrist pull, and awkward kerbs provide a similar experience to the next exercise.

Caution

★ If you experience any pain during this exercise, omit the forward movement, but spend time on all-fours. If the pain persists, stop.

★ If your wrists are painful as a result of this exercise, keep your body weight evenly distributed between your knees and hands. If the pain persists, stop and do more Wrist Curls (see page 62).

1 Kneel on all-fours with your wrists directly under your shoulders, your fingers facing forward, your knees and feet slightly apart, and your knees above your hips. Check your pelvic tilt and tighten your abdominals. Move your body and hips slightly forward, so that most of your body weight is over your wrists.

Ensure the back of your neck is long and in line with your spine

2 Making small, controlled movements, walk your hands forward as far as you can without over-arching your back or moving your knees or feet. Hold, then walk your hands back to the start position. Rest, then repeat.

Do not lock your elbows

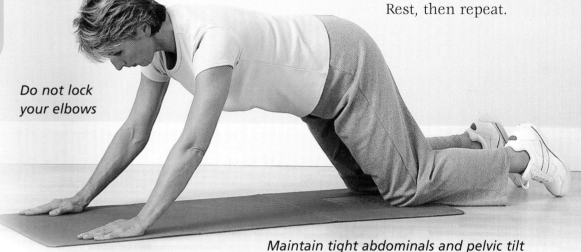

Maintain tight abdominals and pelvic tilt

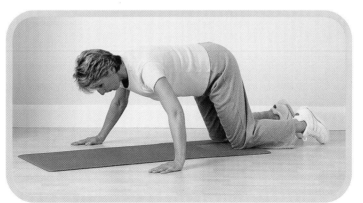

3 Walk your hands out to either side, as far as you can, keeping your body rigid. Hold, then walk your hands back to the start position. Rest, then repeat.

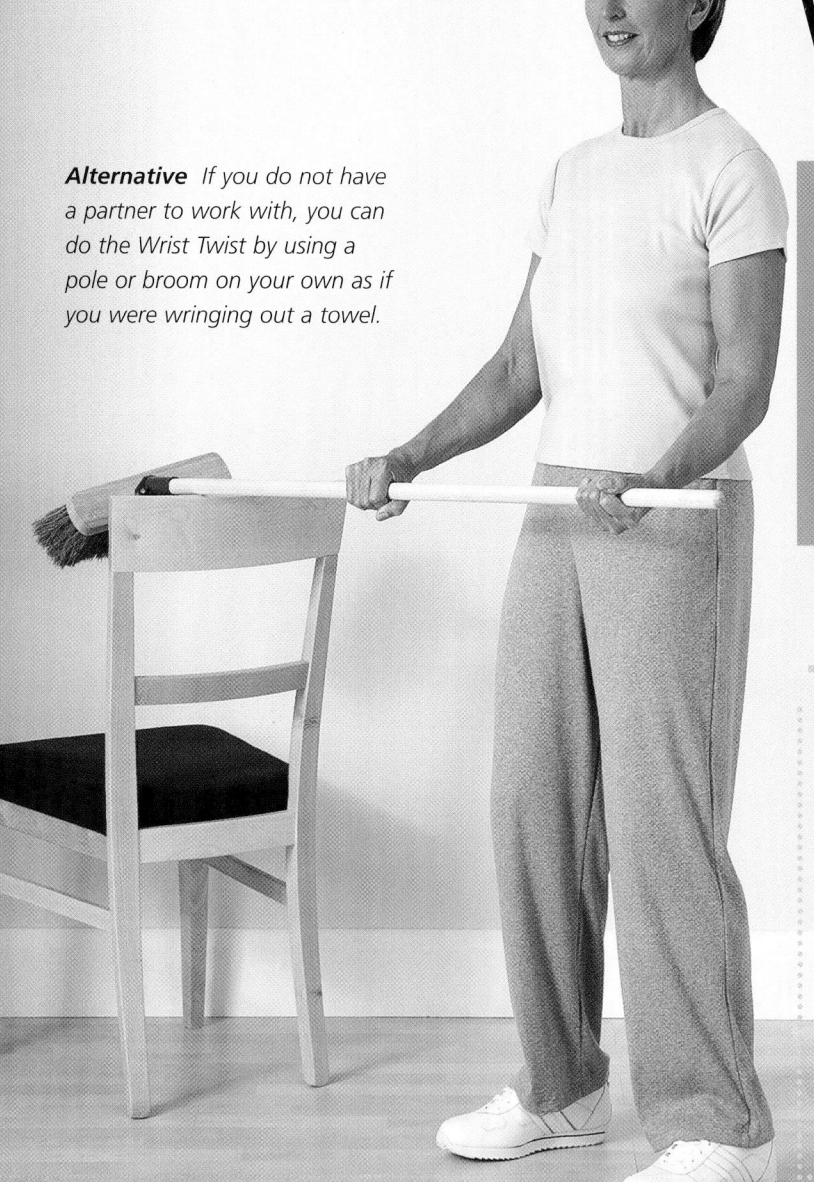

Alternative *If you do not have a partner to work with, you can do the Wrist Twist by using a pole or broom on your own as if you were wringing out a towel.*

Wrist press, twist, & pull

Purpose

To increase bone mineral density (BMD) in the wrists. It also strengthens muscles in the trunk, shoulders, and forearms.

Caution

★ Avoid being competitive, keep the pole equidistant between both partners.

★ If you have arthritis in your hands, do not do this exercise.

These exercises target the muscles controlling the movement of your hands: the wrist flexors and extensors. These are the muscles you use to grip and twist bottle tops, wring wet towels, and push a shopping cart. They load your wrist bone in many directions. You'll need a partner, preferably of a similar size to yourself. If you have to rely on someone bigger, make sure they adjust their strength to meet yours. Use a smooth pole, at least two foot long, such as a body-bar or broom handle. If you cannot find a pole, you could do some arm wrestling at the kitchen table.

There are three exercises here: the press, the twist, and the pull. In each exercise, your partner will be working against you, thus generating high resistant forces. You should feel these forces all the way down your body, proving how many muscle groups are being challenged.

Progression

Generate as much force as you can, counting to three as you press, twist, or pull. Hold for a second before you release.

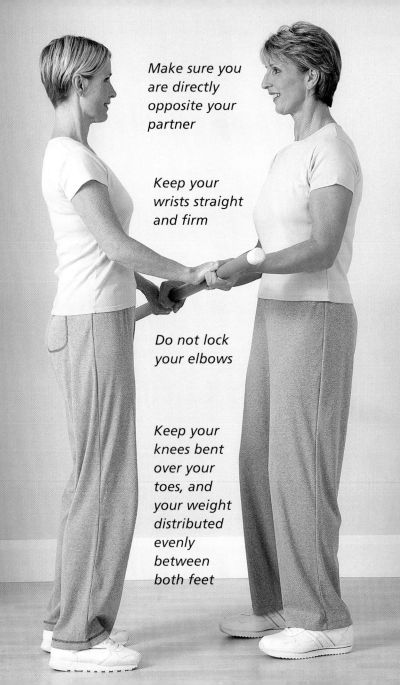

Make sure you are directly opposite your partner

Keep your wrists straight and firm

Do not lock your elbows

Keep your knees bent over your toes, and your weight distributed evenly between both feet

1 **Start** Stand opposite your partner with your feet slightly wider than hip-width apart, and your knees bent. Hold the bar with both hands shoulder-width apart, one hand using an underhand grip, the other over-hand. Check your pelvic tilt and tighten your abdominals.

2 **Press** Push upward with your underhand palm and downward with the other as if trying to rotate the ends of the pole. Your partner should press in the opposite direction. Change your grips around and repeat in the opposite direction. Rest, then repeat.

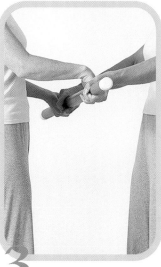

3 **Twist** Return to your start position. Twist the pole, as if wringing a towel. Your partner should twist in the opposite direction. Change your grips and repeat the exercise in the opposite direction. Rest, then repeat.

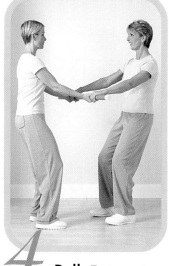

4 **Pull** Return to your start position. Hold the pole with an underhand grip, while your partner uses an overhand grip. Pull in toward your waist as your partner pulls in the opposite direction. Reverse your grip and repeat. Rest, then repeat.

Abdominal lift

This exercise targets the muscles that form the front wall of your lower abdomen. These are important muscles as they support your trunk, and indirectly, your back and spine. They need to be strong to perform your bone-loading exercises effectively; all the forces generated by your arms and legs are supported by the center of your body. These muscles are important for maintaining good posture and correct pelvic tilt. Strong abdominals also give you a trim figure and reduce your risk of falls. Slack abdominal muscles allow your middle to bulge outward and can lead to back pain. Focus on tightening the triangle of muscles spreading from your waistline to your pubic bone.

Unsafe exercise

★ Out-dated sit-ups should be avoided because they increase the risk of vertebral fracture.

Advanced alternative *When you have mastered the Abdominal Lift shown below, try this for an extra challenge.*

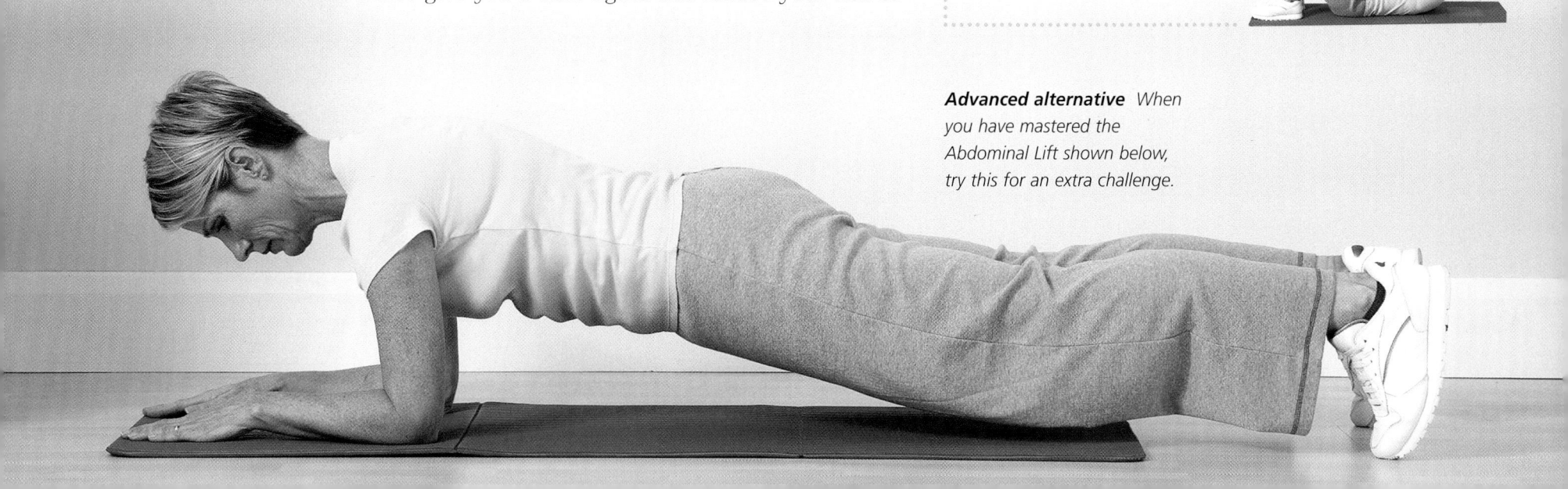

1 Lie face-down with your forehead on your folded hands. Position your legs just a few inches apart. Check your pelvic tilt.

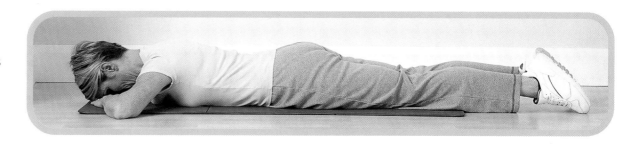

2 Breathe in, then breathe out as you contract your abdominals and lift your navel in toward your spine. Hold, then release back to the start. Rest, then repeat.

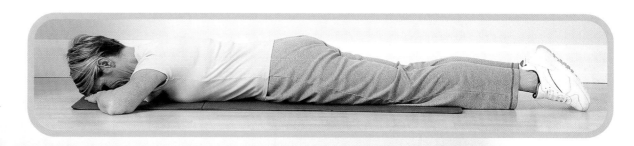

Keep the back of your neck long and your shoulders down

Relax your buttock muscles

3 Progress by positioning your arms, elbows, and shoulders as shown. Lift your navel, abdominals, and hips off the floor. Try not to over-tilt your pelvis. Breathe out as you contract, lift, and pull in. Hold, and breathe in as you release. Rest, then repeat.

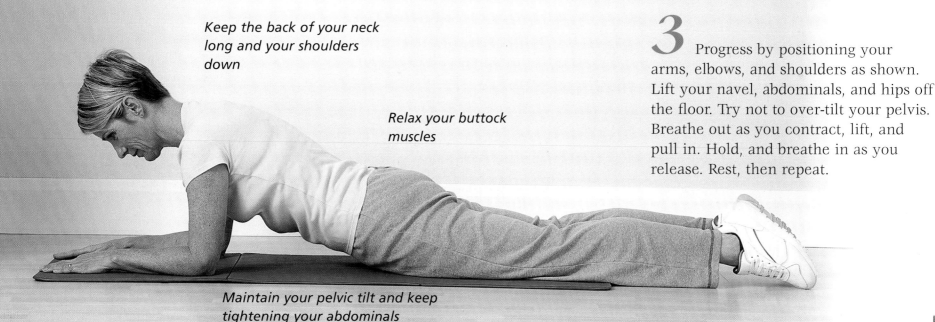

Maintain your pelvic tilt and keep tightening your abdominals

Flexibility stretches

A cool-down using flexibility stretches, gentle relaxation, and brief revitalizing circulation exercises is an essential finish to every exercise program. The exercises have left your muscles warm and pliant, so this is a good time to develop your joint flexibility. Begin by repeating the warm-up stretches (see pages 30–5); the emphasis now should be on developing each stretch as far as you can, comfortably.

Add the two stretches shown here to provide more supported positions for your hamstring and inner thigh muscles. These muscles are especially important to stretch and they respond particularly well to longer, developmental stretches. Extend the duration of the stretches gradually from ten seconds each to one minute.

Purpose

Over time, these stretches will improve your suppleness and reduce the risk of injury in both everyday and recreational activities.

Caution

★ Never bounce in a stretch. This can tighten the muscle you are trying to stretch, and may cause injury.

★ Remain seated a few moments after the lying stretch. Get up slowly to avoid dizziness.

Unsafe exercise

★ Do not touch your toes with straight legs to stretch the back and hamstrings. This outdated stretch carries increased risk of back and eye injuries.

Effective stretching

★ Put on an extra top to retain body heat and to feel more comfortable.

★ It is important to do these longer stretches gradually.

★ Move slowly with control to take your muscles into the fully stretched positions shown.

★ Hold until you feel the tightness subside.

★ Then, on an out-breath, move gently further into the stretch. Try to relax into the stretch.

★ Release any tension in the rest of the body, especially the shoulders.

★ To finish, move slowly out of the stretch again.

Relax and revitalize

★ Spend a few minutes relaxing.

★ Lie on your back on the floor, with knees raised slightly.

★ Tense and relax your muscles to feel the difference in your face, shoulders, hands, all the way down.

★ Do a full body stretch to wake you up again.

★ Revitalize by doing the circulation exercises on page 24.

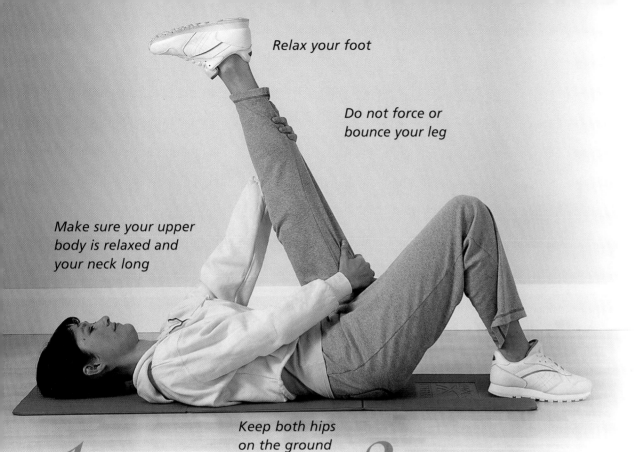

Relax your foot

Do not force or bounce your leg

Make sure your upper body is relaxed and your neck long

Keep both hips on the ground

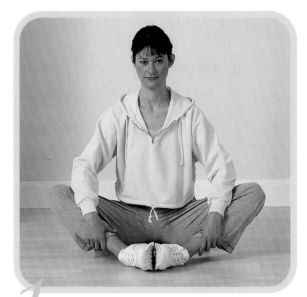

1 **Hamstring stretch** Lie on your back with both knees bent and your feet flat on the floor. Check your pelvic tilt, tighten your abdominals, and, keeping the knee bent, lift one leg in toward your chest. Take hold of the back of your thigh with both hands. Relax for a count of 10.

2 Slowly straighten your leg until you feel a stretch in the back of your raised thigh. Slide your outside hand up onto the lower leg so your whole leg is supported. If you feel the stretch subside, bring the leg gently a little further toward your chest. Hold for a count of 10 or more. Relax, then return to the start and repeat on the other leg.

1 **Inner thigh stretch** Sit on a folded mat with the soles of your feet together, your back long, and your chest lifted. Place your arms on your legs as shown, and allow your knees to open naturally. Check your pelvic tilt and tighten your abdominals.

2 Use your forearms and then your hands to press your legs down gently, until you feel a stretch along your inner thighs. If you feel the stretch subside, lean forward slightly for a deeper stretch. Hold for a count of 10 or more.

Activities for life

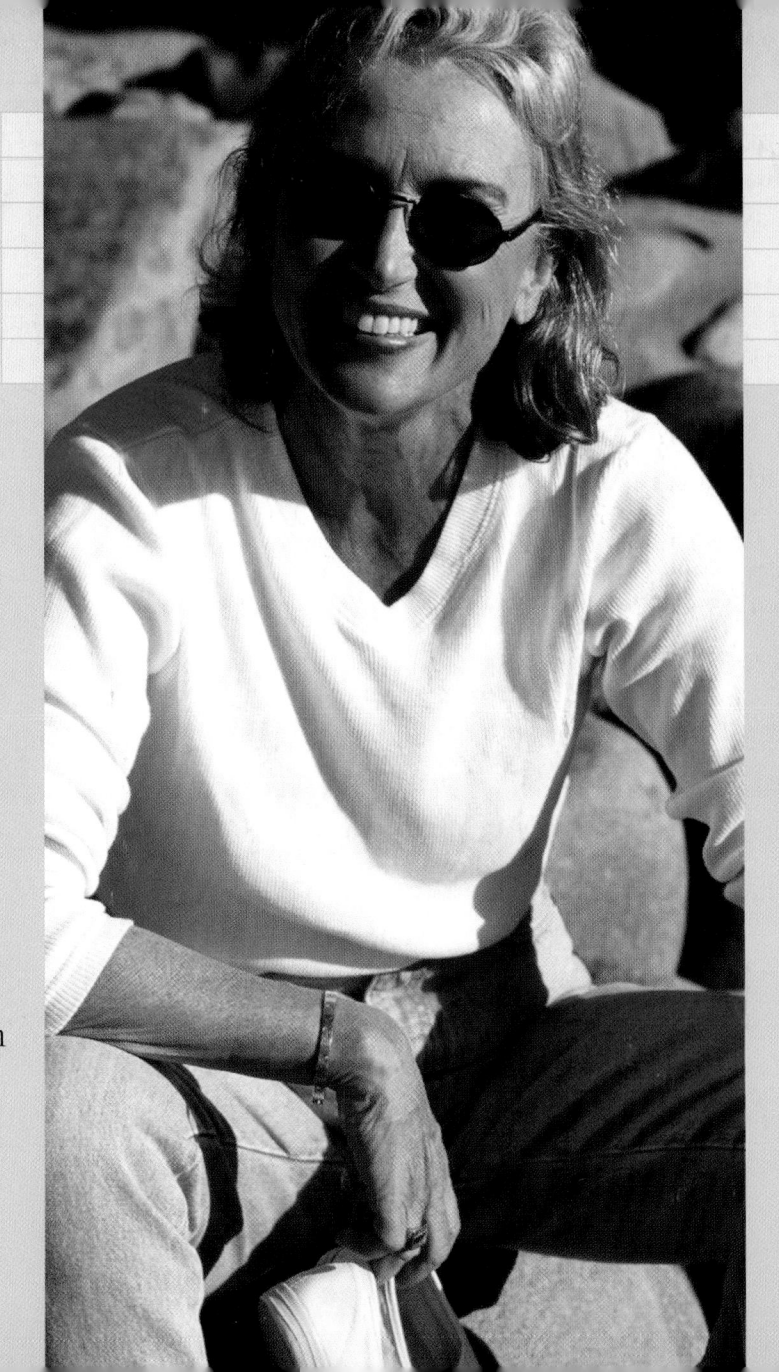

This section contains physical activities for increasing bone strength that you can include in your daily life, both inside and outside of the home. They are weight-bearing activities, which means that you are on your legs and your skeleton is supporting the weight of your body. While these exercises are beneficial for your hips and spine, they won't benefit your wrist bones. Weight-bearing is not the same as weight-training, which is about lifting weights to increase muscle and bone strength.

The exercises in this chapter are arranged in order of increasing intensity. If you have not been exercising regularly before now, start by introducing some gentle activities into your life such as those on pages 81–7. If you are young, healthy, and already lead an active life, the higher-impact exercises on pages 88–91 will further improve your bone strength.

Walking

If you are not in the habit of taking any exercise at all, then a brief daily walk outside the home is a good start. Most people achieve this every day, without thinking of it as exercise at all, but if you are a person who drives everywhere in the car, it is worth adding up how much walking you have done in the last few days.

Women who walk more than one mile a week (that is, about three minutes of walking a day, on average), have a significantly higher BMD than those who walk less than that. Walking for longer periods makes no further difference to BMD, although it has many other health benefits. Other research has shown that women who habitually walk briskly have better BMD than those who tend to walk at a slower rate. It is better, therefore, to take regular short walks than long ones, and to concentrate on walking faster.

Hiking in the countryside is great exercise and is likely to be good for your BMD and balance. The changing gradients and surfaces give a variety of stimulation for bones. As yet, however, there have been no formal studies on the benefits.

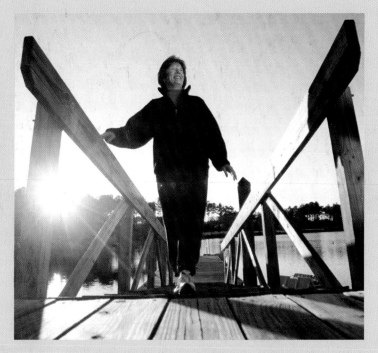

Setting the pace With the help of a car odometer or an accurate map, plan out a quarter of a mile walk near your home or work. If you can walk the distance in five minutes, you are walking at a moderate pace. Aim to improve your time, and try to maintain this pace when walking elsewhere.

Getting started

★ Go for a brisk walk—at least five minutes long—every day.

★ Once you are warmed up, introduce some short spurts of a faster pace for a few seconds, reverting to your chosen speed in between. You should be breathing more than normal, but not breathless.

★ Walking for more than 10 minutes every day does not improve bone health any further, but walk–jog does, so if you can, follow the walk–jog program instead (see pages 84–5).

★ Walking for half an hour once a week is not the same as five minutes daily. Little and often is the way to better bones.

Stair climbing

If you live in a house with stairs you will be giving your leg muscles and skeleton a good daily workout without even realizing it. Climbing stairs is an easy way to increase your daily activity level, and seems to be associated with good BMD and a low risk of fracture. Whenever possible, take the stairs instead of the escalator in a department store or public building, and instead of the elevator in your work place or apartment block. If you live or work in a high-rise, get out of the elevator a story earlier, and walk the rest of the way.

You should aim to climb ten flights of ten stairs per day. If you live in a home with stairs, you will meet this target without even thinking about it. But if you live in a one-story home, then try to take the stairs whenever you are out and about.

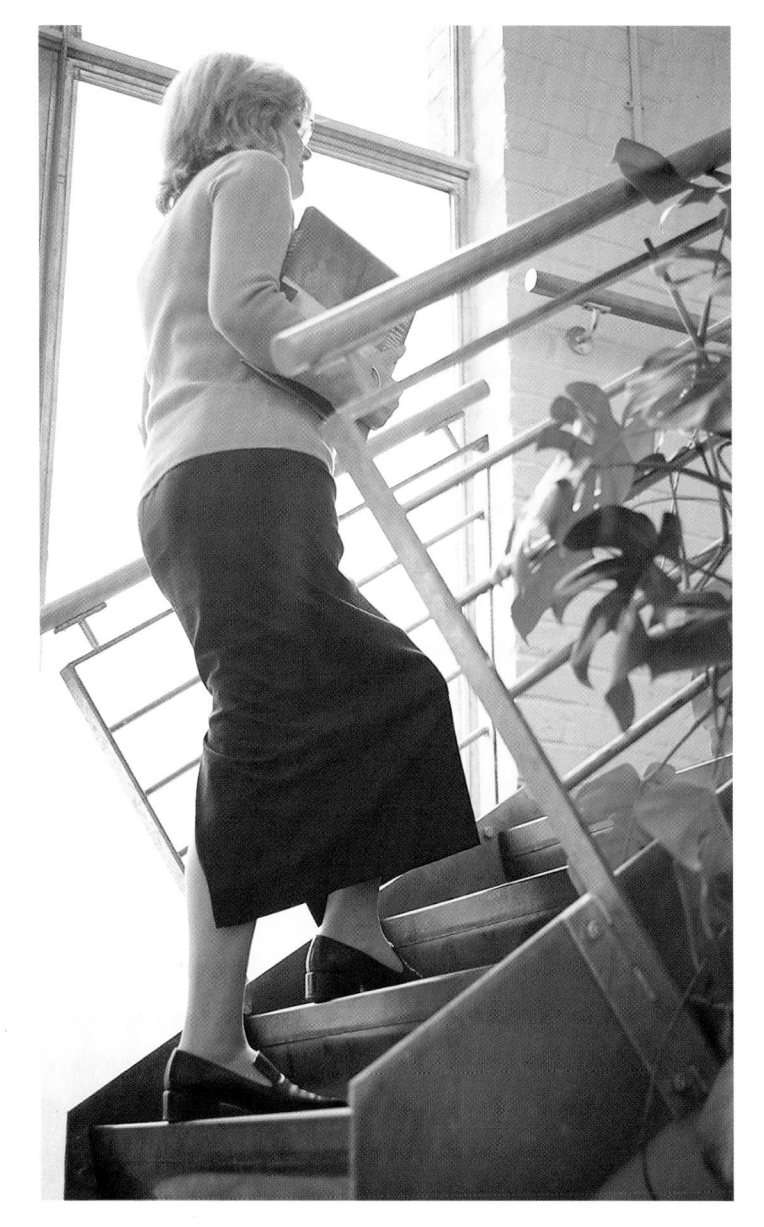

Climb some stairs everyday *This is very good for your bones and the muscle power in your legs. Take the stairs instead of an elevator whenever possible.*

Aquarobics

T'ai Chi Ch'uan

Exercise classes that take place in water, such as aquarobics, use the resistance of the water to develop endurance, muscle strength, flexibility, and balance. Any exercise that improves balance is important for reducing the risk of falls; it is especially helpful for people who have suffered a fall already, and are fearful of falling again. You can work your body hard in the pool without risk, because you are cushioned by the water.

Swimming pool exercise class
This is more fun than swimming lengths, and is very good for improving strength, flexibility, and balance.

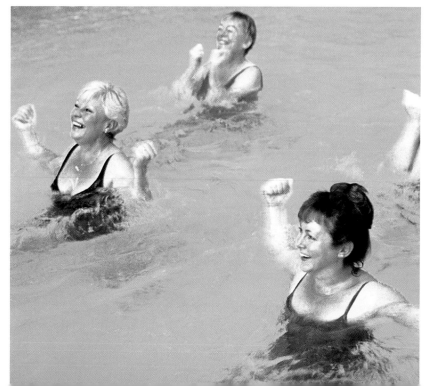

Also known as "T'ai Chi," this ancient practice is an excellent way to develop good balance and strong legs. It also instils a feeling of calmness, peace of mind, and stability. It can be practiced by people of all ages, and is a confidence-booster for those who have suffered a fall.

T'ai Chi originated in China nearly 2000 years BC. It embraces a whole philosophy of life which has its roots in martial arts. It is also a meditative form of weight-bearing exercise which has been adapted to meet the demands and pace of modern life in the West. Balance, power, and energy are the fundamental principles behind T'ai Chi.

It takes a long time to learn T'ai Chi properly, and you need to join a class to do so. Once learned, however, it can be practiced independently.

Walk–jog

Caution

★ Do not jog if the ground is icy, nor if the weather is extremely cold or hot.

★ If you have asthma or are at risk from heart disease or falls, start with a regular walking program for 12 weeks. Make sure you do not get breathless.

This is brisk walking interspersed with a bit of jogging (not to be confused with running, which is much more energetic). Jogging is a much gentler activity than running, with a wide range of energy options. It used to be called "Scout's pace" and it is a very efficient way of getting somewhere quickly without getting too hot, tired, or breathless. Walk–jog can start as a bouncy walk and get more energetic as you improve.

This walk–jog program has been proven to increase BMD in the spine and hips. It needs to be done three times a week in order to be effective, unless you already do other exercise. It should be done on non-consecutive days. Each session should last for about 20 minutes. It doesn't matter where you exercise; it could be in the park, while walking to the mail box, or to work. Wear sensible shoes and comfortable clothes and observe the "Getting started" guidelines on pages 18 and 88.

A walk–jog This activity can be started gently and built up gradually into a useful bone-loading exercise. It is suitable for those unaccustomed to regular exercise.

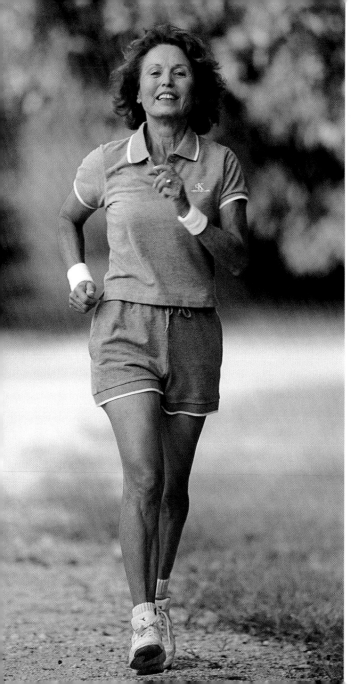

Progression

If you are not used to exercise, start with Stage 1 below. If you are already a frequent brisk walker, start at Stage 2. If you already go jogging or running on a regular basis, consider some weight-training (see page 86).

(see page 86)

Caution

★ If you have arthritis, any leg or back pain, or a diagnosis of osteoporosis, then do not jog. Stick to a daily brisk short walk.

★ If you experience pain of any sort, slow down, or stop.

Stage 1	Stage 2	Stage 3	Stage 4
months 1–2	months 3–4	months 5–6	month 7 onward
★ Brisk walking only, for about 20 minutes	★ Introduce 6 jogging steps after every 60 walking steps	★ Increase your ratio of jogging to walking until you are doing about half and half, say walking for about half a minute, and jogging for half a minute	★ Increase your ratio of jogging to walking until you are walking for half a minute and jogging for a whole minute
★ Try to increase your speed each day	★ If you get hot or breathless, go back to walking for a few minutes, before starting again		★ If you get too hot or breathless, do a bit more walking and a bit less jogging
★ Follow the same route and time yourself			
★ Keep a record in your diary			

Weight-training

This is widely practiced in gyms, sports clubs, and healthclubs. In these settings weight-training is done using free weights as in the home exercises and also using weight-training machines. These machines contain stacks of weights that you raise and lower with your arms or legs using pulleys. Women of all ages do weight-training; you do not have to be strong.

An advantage of using weight-training machines in a gym environment is that there are different machines that allow you to exercise all the major muscle groups in the body. The machines are safe because your back is supported, the start position can be adjusted to suit you, and the weights are within a cage so they cannot do any damage if you let them go.

Weight-training is often confused with weight-lifting which is a competitive sport in which very heavy weights are lifted, and bulging muscles are developed. It has

nothing to do with the particular kind of training recommended in this book; muscles can get much stronger without becoming bulky.

Weight-training can be practiced using small weights and many lifts; this is good for endurance but it does not improve BMD. To improve BMD you need to lift heavier weights quite slowly, a few times. It is important to work up to the heavier weights over several months so you do not injure yourself. Injuries, if they occur, are usually the result of "too much, too soon" or poor technique.

If you have never done any weight-training, seek advice from a qualified instructor about technique and about how the machines work. Most gyms have free introductory sessions, so you can look until you find a gym that suits you. For improvements, train three times a week.

Caution

★ Every woman is different, so it is important that you use a weight that is right for you. Follow the 1RM rule (see Progression below). If in doubt about the most suitable weight to use, seek advice from a qualified instructor.

Devise a gym program

Explain to the gym instructor that you are working to improve your BMD. Ask for a program that includes the following lifts:

Lower body	Upper body
★ hip extension	★ lateral pull down
★ hip flexion	★ bench press
★ hip adduction	★ bicep curl
★ hip abduction	★ back extension
★ leg extension	
★ leg press	

Progression

When you have practiced correct lifting using a weight-training machine at least three times a week for one month, measure your "one repetition maximum" (1RM). Lift a succession of weights once each, resting in between lifts. Increase the weight until you can no longer lift it once with acceptable form. This means smoothly, and steadily through the movement, without any wobbles. The heaviest weight you can lift once is your 1RM. To train effectively for improving BMD, choose weights which are at least 70 percent of your 1RM and do up to eight repetitions. If you can do more, then you need to use a heavier weight. As you improve and can complete eight repetitions easily, use a heavier weight. You should feel that the last lift of the last set is as much as you can manage.

Go to the gym *When you have mastered the exercises contained in this book, you can take your program further by using weight machines in a gym. This woman is doing a leg extension.*

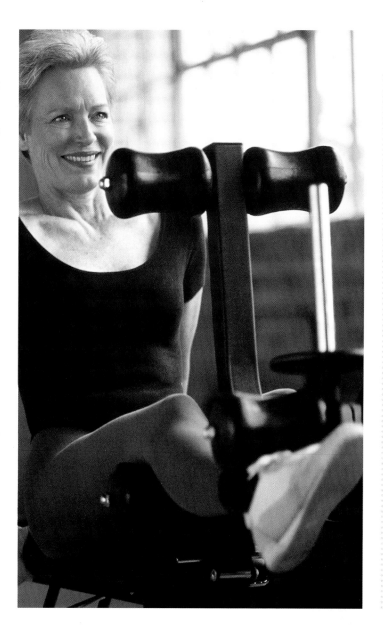

Good technique

★ It is essential to start with light weights that you can lift easily until you have mastered the technique.

★ Make sure that your position is comfortable. Your back should be supported, and your posture should be correct throughout.

★ Lift and lower the weight slowly. Count to three as you lift, and to three as you lower. Rest briefly before the next lift.

★ Breathe evenly throughout while counting out loud. You should not get breathless at any time.

★ Aim for eight lifts, resting for a second between each.

★ Aim to repeat your set of eight lifts twice more, resting for a minute between each set.

★ Remember to warm up first, and stretch afterward.

Jumping

The exercises on the next four pages improve your BMD because of the impacts involved when your feet hit the ground, but they carry a far higher risk of injury than the exercises contained in the main program. Provided they are not practiced to excess, they are recommended for healthy, premenopausal women.

Jumping is an energetic form of exercise, but it only takes a few minutes and you do not have to do many jumps to benefit your bones. It improves BMD in the hips (but not the spine) in premenopausal women, but unfortunately has no effect in postmenopausal women, even if they are taking HRT. Jumping also increases the power in your thighs and calves, and improves your balance.

Caution

★ Jumping is not recommended for women (even premenopausal women) who have poor balance, a history of falls or osteoarthritis in the back, legs, or hips, or a history of pain.

Getting Started

★ You will need to wear supportive shoes with cushioned, flexible shoes (e.g. trainers) to avoid joint injury. You will get warm, so wear comfortable, cotton clothes, and drink water before and afterward.

★ Warm up following the exercises on pages 22–35. It is very important that you feel warm, loose, and relaxed before you start this exercise.

Variation

If you prefer, jump using a rope. This activity is also good for shoulder flexibility and balance.

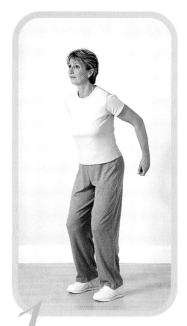

1 Find a well-ventilated space with a firm floor. Stand tall with your feet a hip-width apart. Adjust your pelvic tilt, and let your ankles, knees, and hips give slightly. Bend your knees and swing your arms back to start.

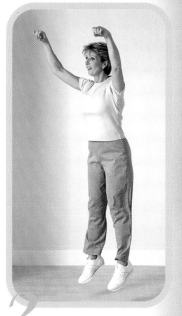

2 Swing your arms forward, and jump into the air with both feet. Aim to jump about 3 inches high—no more. The jump should be done in one smooth, quick movement.

3 Bend your knees as you land. Repeat according to the program opposite.

Look forward

Keep your chest lifted

Land toe–ball–heel

Let your heels land with an audible thump

Progression

★ **Day 1** Start with a few experimental jumps

★ **Day 2** 5 jumps

★ **Day 3** 10 jumps

★ **Day 4** 20 jumps

★ **Day 5** 30 jumps

★ **Day 6** 50 jumps

★ **Day 7** Rest

NOTE: When doing 20 or more jumps, rest between each block of 10 by doing gentle stepping movements.

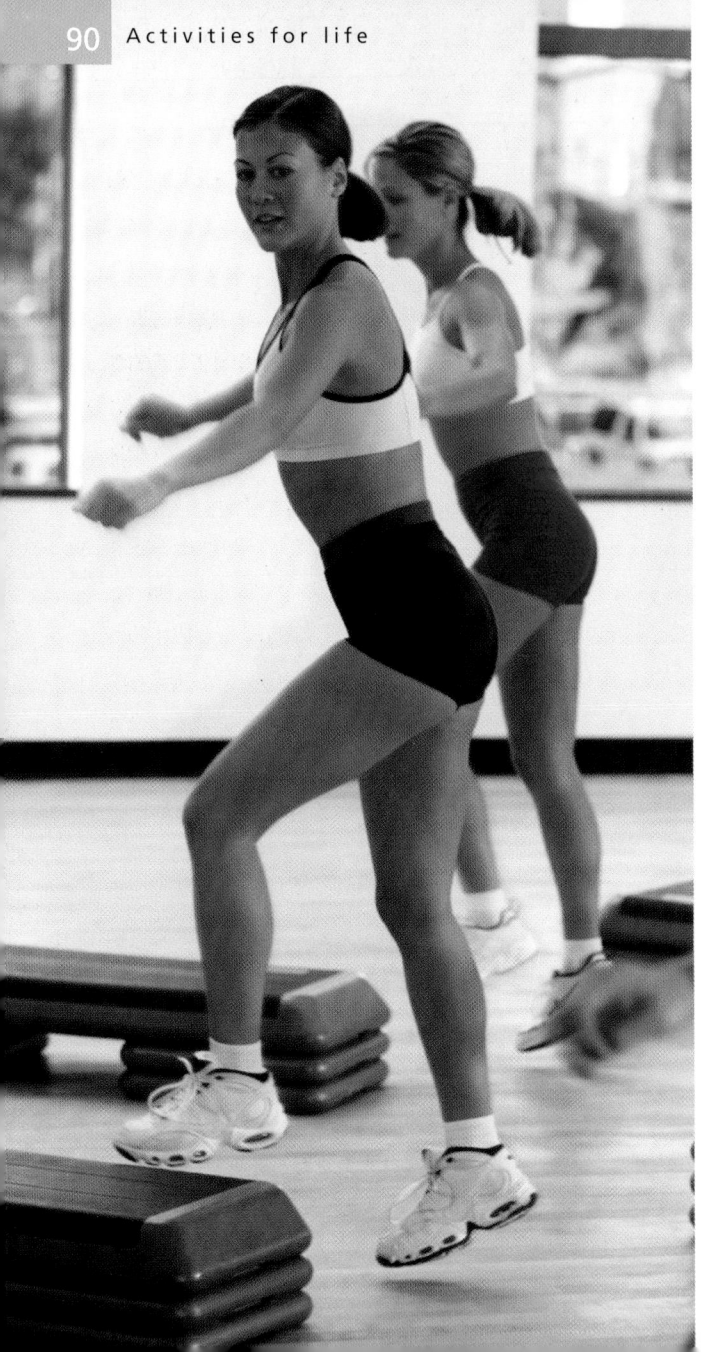

Studio classes

Check your local community for exercise to music classes. They come in many forms and contain a variety of exercises. This variety is useful for bones as it loads the skeleton in lots of different ways. Aerobics classes and circuit-training include weight-bearing exercises, and the best of these include both high- and low-impact work.

It is important to go to the class regularly, three times a week, unless you plan to include other forms of bone-loading activities in your weekly routine.

Power step *This is a vigorous exercise that adds some jumping to stair climbing, so it is likely to load the hips and spine.*

Caution

★ High-impact exercises carry a relatively high risk of injury. They are recommended only for premenopausal women.

Dancing

Since jumping and jogging are both good bone-loaders, it is likely that any dance that involves ground impact will have the same effect. Tap, Scottish, and Irish dancing should all be effective.

Gentler forms of dance such as line dancing or ballroom dancing are very good for maintaining or improving balance, but they are unlikely to stimulate your bones.

Active sports

Any sport that involves impact is likely to benefit your bones. Racquet sports such as tennis or squash should be effective, as will any sport that involves running and jumping, such as basketball.

Swimming and cycling, although very good for your health in other ways, are not effective for improving BMD.

Running

There is good evidence from studies in the USA that running stimulates BMD at both the spine and the hip in young women aged 20 years.

The usual recommendation is to run for 20–30 minutes, three times a week. This works well for reducing the risk of coronary heart disease and related problems. But there is evidence that shorter periods of running might do your skeleton just as much good.

In 20 minutes of running or jogging, your leading foot hits the ground at least 2000 times. However, fewer impacts are known to be effective for bone, so you may prefer to opt for intermittent jogging instead (see page 84).

Asphalt or grass are better running surfaces for your joints than hard concrete. Wear light-colored clothes if you go running in traffic, for safety.

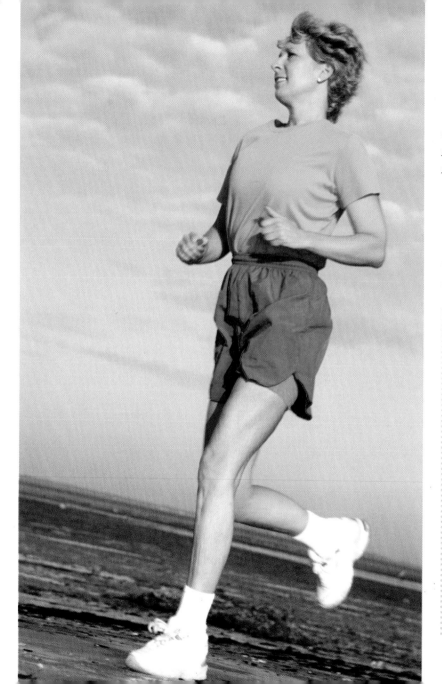

Go for a run *It will load your skeleton and it only needs a short run to be effective.*

Caution

★ Jogging or running for long periods on hard surfaces increases the risk of osteoarthritis and should be avoided if you are vulnerable to this disease.

★ You will need to wear supportive shoes with cushioned, flexible shoes (e.g. trainers) to avoid joint injury. You will get warm, so wear comfortable, cotton clothes, and drink water before and afterward.

Health questionnaire

Ask yourself the following questions	If your answer is YES
★ Have you been in hospital in the last six months? ★ Have you had any major illness or surgery in the last six months? ★ Do you have any current health problems for which you are under active treatment with medication, radiation, or surgery? ★ Have you had a blackout or fallen more than twice in the past year?	Consult with your doctor about starting this new exercise program. Take the book with you to show him what you want to do.
★ Do you have asthma or heart disease? ★ Do you get pain in your chest, neck, or arm when exercising which does not go away when you rest for a few minutes?	Use your prescribed medication and avoid getting breathless, and avoid jumping or jogging unless you are used to doing this.
★ Do you have high blood pressure or are you on treatment for it?	Limit any lift or muscle effort to five seconds.
★ Do you have an artificial hip?	Look for special advice in caution boxes.
★ Do you have tendonitis, bursitis, or rheumatoid arthritis?	Avoid exercises which involve affected parts of your body.
★ Do you have any abnormalities or pain when you walk such as a limp, painful joints, or bunions? ★ Do you have chronic pain in your knees?	Avoid jogging or jumping and use seated alternatives of the home exercises.
★ Do you have chronic pain in your hips or back? ★ Have you been diagnosed as osteoporotic (see below)? ★ Have you fallen once or twice in the past year? ★ Do you have poor balance or poor coordination?	Avoid jogging or jumping; use seated alternatives of the home exercises; limit weights to 10 lbs; avoid the Shoulder Press exercise; and prioritize the Back Lift, Shoulder Mobilizer, Chest Stretch, and balance exercises

Health problems and exercise

If you can answer "no" honestly to all the questions above, then all the home exercises should be safe for you, but if you are in any doubt, consult your doctor. If you have answered "yes" to any question, follow the advice in the right-hand column and observe caution boxes.

Osteoporosis

The diagnosis of osteoporosis is usually made when a bone scan using dual-energy X-ray absorptiometry (DXA) results in a "T score" of 2.5 or more below normal values, when a bone fracture occurs with minimal impact (low trauma), or there are several risk factors (see page 8). Diagnoses based on Ultrasound need to be confirmed with DXA. A diagnosis of "osteopenia," means you have a lower than normal BMD but you are not osteoporotic.

This book is designed to reduce the risk of developing osteoporosis but if you already have this problem the exercise prescription must be modified. For example, high impact exercise is more likely to harm than help because it could cause a fracture. You need to concentrate on the good practice section and the balance exercises in order to protect you against falls, and the home exercises for your back in order to strengthen the supporting muscles round your spine and to help you to keep your spine straight.

Osteoarthritis

This disease is often confused with osteoporosis because the names are similar; it is a disease of the joints, not the bones, from which many women suffer in later life.

The symptoms are pain at night and stiffness in the morning, typically affecting the hands, knees, and hips. Impact loads must be avoided, and exercise which is free of joint loading, such as swimming, is most beneficial.

The gentle options of the home exercises will maintain muscle strength around the joint and help to control pain, and stretching is useful for improving joint function and range of movement.

Cardiovascular problems

Heart disease is common in later life but the home exercises are not designed to cause breathlessness, high pulse rates, or raised blood pressure. If you do the gentle options slowly, with rests as prescribed on page 37, and pay attention to the cautions with each exercise, there should be no cardio-respiratory distress.

Falls

These are also common in later life and are the main cause of fractures, so if you have a history of falls avoid exercises which put you at risk. The good practice, balance, and home exercises should safely improve your postural control.

Physical activity checklist

These questions are to help you check out both your present activity levels, and what you are currently able to do. Answering them honestly will enable you to identify those areas needing improvement, and to tailor an exercise program which is relevant for you. Find out how to test yourself safely by looking up the page numbers listed.

What was your score?

★ You are safe to do all the home exercises if you scored 25 or over in "Did you," and 40 or over in "Can you."

★ If your scores were below this, choose the gentler versions of the exercises and progress slowly.

★ If your score was below 7 in "Did you," and below 15 in "Can you," then start with the good practice section, balance exercises, walking, stair climbing, and aquarobics.

Did you..?

	Score
★ Yesterday did you walk anywhere...	
at a brisk pace?	3
at a normal pace?	1
at a slow pace?	0
★ Yesterday, did you walk for over 5 minutes?	3
★ Yesterday, did you climb 5 flights of stairs?	4
★ During the last week did you . . .	
go to a gym?	5
attend an exercise class?	5
play any other sport?	5
take any other exercise?	5

Only score here if your activities were bone-loading (see Activities for life page 80)

Note your score and chart your improvements

DATE   TOTAL SCORE =

Can you..?

	Score
★ Can you balance on one leg for 30 seconds? (see page 38)	5
★ Can you reach the back of your neck? (see page 34)	5
★ Can you walk on your toes for 20 steps? (see page 42)	5
★ Can you walk for 5 minutes at 4 mph? (see page 81)	5
★ Can you jog for 5 minutes at 5 mph? (see page 84)	10
★ Can you raise your head 4 inches off the floor in a back lift? (see page 44)	5
★ Can you do 16 side leg lifts? (see page 50)	5
★ Can you lift 3 lbs in a wrist curl? (see page 62)	5

Note your score and chart your improvements

DATE   TOTAL SCORE =

Tailor your own program

There are more exercises in the book than you could complete in one session so choose the ones which will be most useful to you, and vary them from time to time.

Each exercise takes about 5 minutes for 3 sets of 8 lifts, and the double exercises (left + right side) take about 6 minutes, so you can do 6 single or 4 double exercises in a 40 minute session, in addition to preparation, warm-up, stretching, and relaxing. Later on, you can fit in more exercises by combining them (see "For experienced exercisers"). Here are some ideas to help you plan. Don't forget your daily half dozen (see pages 18–21).

Planning your session

Always include these elements:
* Prepare your space and warm-up
* Balance exercises
* Home exercises
* Stretch and relax

For beginners or older women

Begin with these 8 home exercises which do not need any equipment. Add a few new ones week by week.

* **Monday**   Back Lift
                                    Side Leg Lift
                                    Arm Press
                                    Straight Leg Lift

* **Wednesday**   Aquarobics or T'ai Chi

* **Friday**   Leg Lift
                                    Abdominal Lift
                                    All-fours
                                    Thigh Lift

OR

On three separated days of the week, work through the stages of the walk–jog program (see page 84) and do the Wrist Press, Twist, & Pull exercises (see page 74). Take a stout walking stick and a friend and do it all in the park.

For experienced exercisers

You can save time during your workout by combining exercises which use different muscle groups instead of resting between sets. For example, combine the Flying Back Lift and Chest Press:

* **Flying Back Lift**
  Do 8 lifts, roll over, then pick up dumbbells
* **Chest Press**
  Do 8 lifts, put down dumbbells, and roll over to do Flying Back Lifts again.

For double exercises, do 16 lifts (left + right side) of the first exercise then change over.

Other good pairings are:
* Shoulder Press + Arm Curl
* Back Lift + All-fours
* Abdominal Lift + Leg Lift
* Straight Leg Lift + Standing Leg Curl
* Thigh Lift + Leg Press

Index

Useful addresses

National Osteoporosis Foundation (N.O.F.)
1232 22nd St. N.W., Washington D.C. 20037–1292, (202) 223–2226

SPRI Products Inc. (Rubber resistance exercise products)
1026 Campus Drive, Mundelein, IL 60060, (800) 222–7774

Cybex (Cardiovascular and strength equipment)
10 Trotter Drive, Medway, MA 02053–2299, (888) 462–9239

Life Fitness Inc. (Exercise equipment)
10601 W. Belmont Avenue, Franklin Park, IL 60131, (800) 634–8637

References

▨ E. Bassey, M. Rothwell et al. *Pre- and postmenopausal women have different bone mineral density responses to the same high-impact exercise.* J Bone Miner Res 1998; 13:1805–13.

▨ C. Coupland, S. Cliffe et al. *Habitual physical activity and bone mineral density in postmenopausal women in England.* Int J Epidemiol 1999; 28:241–6.

▨ D. Kerr, A. Morton et al. *Exercise effects on bone mass are site-specific and load dependent.* J Bone Miner Res 1996; 11:218–25.

▨ W. Kohrt, D. Snead et al. *Additive effects of weight-bearing exercise and estrogen on bone mineral density in older women.* J Bone Miner Res 1995; 10:1303–11.

▨ E. A. Krall, B. Dawson-Hughes. *Walking is related to bone density and rates of bone loss.* Am J Med 1994; 96:20–6.

▨ T. Lohman, S. Going et al. *Effects of resistance training on regional and total bone mineral density in premenopausal women: A randomized prospective study.* J Bone Miner Res 1995; 10:1015–24.

▨ M. Revel, M. Mayou-Benhamou et al. *One-year psoas training can prevent lumbar bone loss in postmenopausal women: a randomised controlled trial.* Calcif Tissue Int 1993; 53:307–11.

▨ M. Sinaki, B. A. Mikkelsen. *Postmenopausal spinal osteoporosis: flexion versus extension exercises.* Arch Phys Med Rehabil 1984; 65:593–6.

▨ C. Snow-Harter, M. L. Bouxsein et al. *Effects of resistance and endurance exercise on BM status of young women: a randomized exercise intervention trial.* J Bone Miner Res 1992; 7:761 –9.

▨ L. Welsh, O. M. Rutherford. *Hip bone mineral density is improved by high-impact aerobic exercise in postmenopausal women and men over 50 years.* Eur J Appl Physiol 1996; 74:511–7.